Do You Have Two Weeks?
That's all you need to...
Drop Pounds. Lose Inches. Get Gorgeous.

"It takes a lot to motivate me to exercise, but Physique 57 is the ideal workout. It's efficient, fun, and targeted to get the results you didn't think were possible!"

—Demi Moore

"In just two weeks I fit into my jeans from high school."   —Parker Posey

"The *most* efficient workout I've ever done—and let me tell you, I've done them *all*!"   —Lisa Rinna

"I really enjoy the Physique 57 workout. It's challenging and the hard work pays off!"   —Denise Richards

"Physique 57 makes exercise fun! A great way to get in shape fast and maintain long, lean muscles. I love it!"   —Lydia Hearst

"This fun workout was transformational; I could see a difference physically within five classes. It changed my life!"   —Kelly Ripa

THE

5*7*

PHYSIQUE®

SOLUTION

**The Groundbreaking 2-Week Plan
for a Lean, Beautiful Body**

TANYA BECKER and
JENNIFER MAANAVI

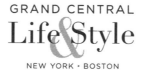
GRAND CENTRAL
Life & Style
NEW YORK · BOSTON

Copyright © 2012 by Jevo Media, Inc.
Photographs by Sara Beth Turner

Grand Central Life & Style
Hachette Book Group
237 Park Avenue
New York, NY 10017
www.GrandCentralLifeandStyle.com

Printed in the United States of America

RRD-C

Originally published in hardcover by Grand Central Life & Style.

First trade edition: January 2013

10 9 8 7 6 5 4 3 2 1

Grand Central Life & Style is an imprint of Grand Central Publishing.

The Grand Central Life & Style name and logo are trademarks of Hachette Book Group, Inc.

The Hachette Speakers Bureau provides a wide range of authors for speaking events. To find out more, go to www.hachettespeakersbureau.com or call (866) 376-6591.

The publisher is not responsible for websites (or their content) that are not owned by the publisher.

The Library of Congress has cataloged the hardcover edition as follows:

Becker, Tanya.
The physique 57 solution : the groundbreaking 2-week plan for a lean, beautiful body /
Tanya Becker and Jennifer Maanavi. — 1st ed.
p. cm.
ISBN 978-0-446-58533-0
1. Reducing exercises.   2. Weight loss.   3. Exercise for women.   I. Maanavi, Jennifer.
II. Title.   III. Title: Physique fifty-seven solution.
RA781.6.B43 2012
613.2'5—dc23
2011017049

ISBN 978-0-446-58534-7 (pbk.)

This book is dedicated to my family for all your love and support, especially my mother, Grace, for being my biggest fan. To Lotte Berk, without your ingenuity I would still be seeking the perfect exercise method. To Jennifer Maanavi, my friend and partner, your talents and zeal constantly amaze me. You are a daily source of inspiration. To Faith, Clark, Sam, and Ted for keeping me present and making sure I stop and enjoy the simple pleasures in life. And to my husband, Terry, for your love, unwavering support, and willingness to walk down any piazza with me.

—Tanya

To Mom, Dad, and Vicky for all the dance lessons and your lifelong support and pride in my success. You've always encouraged me to dance and never sit one out, and for that I am forever grateful. To The Steffi Nossen School of Dance, a great place for a little girl to grow up.

To Tanya Becker for being the perfect artistic force who accepts nothing but victory. For you I push myself harder in class and in life. To Dariush, my love, your intellectual thirst and precision are the spice of our lives. With you, life is exciting and rewarding, and I am obliged to be my best. And to Alec, Halle, and Cameron, your smiling faces and constant giggles make life too good to miss a moment!

—Jennifer

CONTENTS

PART THREE: THE WORKOUTS

PART FOUR: THE MENU

INTRODUCTION

The First Step to a Gorgeous Physique

Hello, Gorgeous!

Welcome to *The Physique 57 Solution*, your own personal prescription for a lean and beautiful body. Starting today, it's time to say good-bye to all the other workouts you've known and tried—the ones that haven't worked for you because they didn't produce results, didn't fit your lifestyle, or were just plain boring. If you've been looking for a so-good-it's-addictive fitness regimen to spark record weight loss and sculpt your body in record time, we're here to tell you that it *does* exist—and that Physique 57 is the program for you!

Committing to a new workout is an empowering choice, and we congratulate you on taking this step. By picking up this book, you are already on your way to achieving the gorgeous physique you've always wanted: no more wasted hours at the gym, no more fretting over extra pounds, no more muffin tops, love handles, jiggling thighs, or flabby arms. Instead, in just two weeks' time, you are going to see remarkable changes in your body from head to toe: smooth and sculpted thighs, a lifted seat, a taut, tucked tummy, and slim and sexy arms. You'll stand taller, feel stronger, and go about your day feeling energized and on top of the world because you will look fabulous—and you'll know it! You'll even be able to break out your skinny jeans again. What could be better than that?

We know that our program gets results because we see it happen with our clients all the time. Every day, tens of thousands of women arrive at our studios or pop in our DVDs and push themselves to the limit because they know that our workouts will give them a better body than any other exercise method around. Our new clients are often thrilled to see new muscle definition after their very first class—welcome back, abs!—or discover that they've dropped a whole dress size after just a few sessions. Regardless of what other diets or exercise plans will tell you, you *can* see dramatic changes in just two weeks. And this blockbuster combination of efficiency and results is what has made Physique 57 today's hottest workout—and keeps our clients coming back for more.

This book, which combines two of our signature 57-minute workouts with our delicious, super-slimming meal plan, puts the power of Physique 57 in your hands. And today marks the start of a whole new you. If you're looking to whip your body into shape for a special event, or simply to boost your strength, energy, and overall health while naturally achieving your ideal weight, our two-week plan will give you the same rapid-results workouts our clients get, along with an amazing array of tasty dishes designed to help you maximize your workouts and melt away the pounds. With our eating plan, you can forget the word *diet*. There's no counting calories, no points, no weekly weigh-ins—just simple, macronutrient-rich meals bursting with flavor that will satisfy your cravings and jump-start your body's own natural weight-loss process. By following our program, you can expect to lose:

- Up to 10 pounds
- 2 inches off your waist
- 2 inches off your hips
- 5 inches off your thighs
- 1 inch off your arms

That said, Physique 57 is NOT about being supermodel-skinny—let's get that out of the way right now. It's about being healthy, being fit, and feeling fabulous whatever you do. Some of our happiest clients are those who have only lost a pound or two, and yet their entire body has changed: inches have disappeared, muffin tops have vanished, and trouble spots have been tightened and sculpted to give them a whole new look.

Our program is designed to accommodate all fitness levels, but it's also designed to keep challenging you so that you never perfect the exercises and you NEVER plateau. You can use this plan far beyond the first two weeks and continue to see amazing results. And as you get leaner and stronger and more comfortable with the moves, you can work more efficiently and target your muscles even more effectively, ultimately achieving the best body you've ever had.

Our Story

Before we created Physique 57, we were two women, just like you, who tried time and again to find the secret to staying fit. Growing up, we were both dancers: Jennifer danced with a ballet company during high school, and Tanya studied dance throughout her school years and later on in New York City. But during our twenties, we also picked up many of the bad habits that go along with city living. Our slim and svelte dancers' bodies started to change, and even Tanya, who continued to dance professionally, saw the numbers on the scale start to creep up. Like most women, we wanted to look better, lose a few pounds, firm up soft spots, and wear a bikini without thinking twice.

We tried all of the usual tactics to get back in shape: joined gyms, attended Spin classes, did step aerobics, and took Pilates. Jennifer even tried running with weights strapped to her ankles (talk about agony!). But nothing ever seemed to work, and even though we'd lose a pound or two with each new effort, the look of our bodies stayed mostly the same. More important, none of these workout methods ever *felt* good or satisfying. They all felt like a chore, something we had to get through. We'd be doing a thousand steps in step class, or sweating away on machines at the gym (there's nothing like grunting and sweating in public to make you feel attractive), and all the while we'd be thinking to ourselves: *This may be burning calories, but it doesn't* feel *good—is this REALLY how women were meant to stay fit?*

During this time, we both came to further appreciate the grace and inherent logic of dance: the way the moves and sequences fit together, and the way that every single movement challenged our muscles through precision and form. As any dancer will tell you, ballet is one of the highest forms of athleticism you can find, yielding strong, supple muscles and a long, lean shape. Yet the only machinery you need is your body. There are no steps, no StairMasters, no clunky weights or strength-training machines—just your own form moving in ways that it has been naturally designed to do. We hadn't danced to get in shape; we danced because we loved it. And until recently, it had been more effective at keeping us fit than any other exercise method. Why couldn't we find a workout that felt like dance?

It was then that we each discovered the Lotte Berk Method®, a highly respected fitness technique created by the legendary Russian ballet dancer Lotte Berk, which had been flourishing among Manhattan's elite for thirty years. Jennifer overheard someone talking about it at a party; Tanya answered an ad in the *Village Voice* that was looking for dancers to teach at the Method's Upper East Side and Hamptons studios. We both tried it and were immediately hooked—Jennifer knew ten minutes into her first class that this was the technique she would do for the rest of her life. Tanya went for her audition and was stunned to discover that even the older women in the classes could outperform her in every way—they were stronger, more flexible, and had more stamina, even though Tanya was a professional dancer. Both of us realized that Berk had hit on something special, and that her Method was something we wanted to learn.

In the months that followed, each of us experienced firsthand the transformative results of Berk's intense strengthening and stretching regimen. Tanya began teaching classes at the Lotte Berk Method, and watched the pounds disappear as her muscles became leaner and stronger than they had ever been in her life. Jennifer began taking classes three or four times a week, and just two months later was astonished when she had to have *all* of her clothes tailored and taken in. Her husband, her friends, and even her Wall Street colleagues began commenting on how, well, *hot* she looked! Walking down the hall at the office, she could actually feel that her muscles were different: tight and strong. Even better, the back pain she'd experienced for nearly ten years disappeared. Plus, we both loved the rush we got from making it through one of the ultra-challenging workouts—we'd feel sore afterward, but also energized and powerful, and that feeling was nothing short of addictive.

But even though we both became regulars at the Lotte Berk Method—Tanya as an instructor and Jennifer as a client—it wasn't until many years later that we actually met. In 2005, the studio regretfully announced that it would be closing its doors. We were crushed, but we also knew there was an opportunity. By that time, Tanya had been a master instructor at the Lotte Berk Method for ten years, and Jennifer, now a long-standing Berk devotee, had earned her MBA and was intrigued by the entrepreneurial possibilities. We both felt that the regimen deserved a much larger following, and that it had the potential to take the fitness world by storm. Jennifer even looked into buying the studio, but wasn't making much headway... until one of the staff members suggested that we meet.

So we did. And from that moment on, we knew that we were at the start of an amazing partnership. We found that we had very similar visions: We wanted to take everything that was great about the Lotte Berk Method and build on it to make it even better. We knew that the foundations of the program were strong, but we also knew that after thirty-some years with minimal changes, it was definitely ripe for a makeover.

Together we set out to create the next incarnation of the technique and bring it to a wider audience. Tanya refined and updated the method to make it even more rigorous and effective by adding a greater variety of exercises, along with more strength- and stamina-building variations. We added other modern touches, set the moves to upbeat music, and streamlined the workout so it could be performed in less than an hour. When we happened to find the perfect studio space on New York City's West 57th Street, the city's main thoroughfare right off glamorous Fifth Avenue, the number seemed to tie everything together—and *voilà*, Physique 57 was born!

We've come a long way since those early days as a small group of teachers based out of a single Manhattan studio. Today we are a bona fide fitness movement with studios in Manhattan, the Hamptons, and Beverly Hills; a booming presence online; celebrity clientele; and a best-selling series of award-winning instructional DVDs. But our promise to you remains the same: No matter what kind of shape you have genetically, whether you loathe the gym or already work out seven days a week, our breakthrough exercise regimen will completely transform your body—and you will love every minute of it.

Are You Ready?

Everything you need to achieve a gorgeous physique—the moves, the meals, and the motivation—is in this book. That said, it's not enough just to read these pages and try out a few of the exercises and recipes. If you want a great body, you have to work for it. No matter what your age or starting point, whether you want to lose five pounds or fifty, what you put in is what you'll get back out. So for these next two weeks, we want you to really *bring it*! Show us how fierce and unstoppable you are with every set of reps, every workout, every food choice, and every decision you make that supports your new, healthier lifestyle. We know you can do it, so take this moment right now to commit to giving this program your all. Put aside any fears, doubts, or excuses, and tap into the part of you that is hardworking, ambitious, and never, ever afraid of a challenge. Yes, many of the moves in our workouts will be new, and YES, we're going to push you to feel the burn and fight through it because that's when the magic happens. But we also know that you're going to love the excitement of the Physique 57 experience: the fun choreography, the energizing pace, and the incredible rush that comes from knowing that even if you're working out harder than you ever have in the past, you CAN do it, and it feels great!

We like to remind our clients at the beginning of every session, "*You* are the sculptor. You are in charge." And it's true: You are the architect of your body, and you have the power to design it any way you want. Together, we are going to chisel, sculpt, and cinch every inch of you to create the physique you've always wanted. So to get going, let's learn a bit more about what makes our workout so effective and unique. Then it's time to wake up those muscles, rev up your metabolism, and start feeling some heat! We can't wait, because we know what lies ahead.

You're going to be amazing. This is your time to shine.

PART ONE

THE METHOD

1

WHAT IS PHYSIQUE 57?

IF YOU'RE ANYTHING LIKE US, YOUR BIGGEST CHALLENGE when it comes to getting fit isn't a lack of interest—and it certainly isn't laziness. On the contrary, if you're like most of the women we know, you are already your own version of Superwoman: hardworking, kind, and capable of juggling dozens of responsibilities and commitments every day. The problem is that everything else on your to-do list often seems far more interesting and enjoyable than exercise. And let's face it—it usually is! After all, who wants to be running to nowhere on a treadmill when you could be out socializing with your friends or playing with your kids?

If this is your first experience with Physique 57, we can promise you that it is like nothing you've ever seen in a gym, and it's far from a typical aerobics or step class. Our workout is designed for maximum effectiveness and efficiency—but it's also designed to be FUN. Most of today's big fitness names and personal trainers use the same techniques and exercises that have been around for decades: a combination of weight training and cardio that includes jogging in place, lunges, squats, side bends, crunches, and all the other classic moves, just rearranged in different combinations. Talk about uninspiring! Our workout, on the other hand, is 100 percent unique: a totally creative sequence of moves designed to keep you challenged, motivated, *and* entertained. We know that the key to sticking with any workout is to enjoy it so much that you and your body actually crave it, because only then will it become a lifestyle.

We also believe that in addition to the moves themselves, the tone and feel of the workout really matter. Many of today's fitness gurus apply the straight-talking, boot-camp-style approach to exercise, and while this might make for great reality television, we prefer a decidedly different approach. Because our program is fundamentally based on classical ballet and the Lotte Berk Method, our workouts retain a sense of grace and femininity. We're all about feeling the burn and pushing ourselves to the limit, but we're also about creating something beautiful: beautiful posture, beautiful movements, and ultimately a beautiful you. We firmly believe that the way you work out determines how you design your body; if you desire a long, lean, sexy shape, your exercise regimen should make you feel like a dancer, not a bodybuilder. Every single minute of our workouts is designed not only to make you stronger, but also to beautify the way you stand, the way you move, and the way you carry yourself in the world each day.

Now that you understand our fitness philosophy, let's take a closer look at the Physique 57 method and how it works.

Our Foundation: The Lotte Berk Method

Physique 57's most important precursor, the Lotte Berk Method, was developed during the 1950s by Russian ballet dancer Lotte Berk. Berk was a London-based, classically trained dancer who had a distinguished career with a prominent dance company until a car accident left her with a serious spinal injury. Working with orthopedic specialists, she began to design a series of exercises based on her own ballet barre routines that would strengthen her spine and core and assist in her rehabilitation. Her aim was to regain her former strength and suppleness, as well as tone and shape her entire musculature, which had weakened substantially during the long months of inactivity.

Berk's strengthening regimen worked so well that she was able to make a full recovery. Soon she began sharing her exercise method with others, and the results she saw in her students led her to open her own studio in 1959. In addition to being rehabilitative, the method seemed to deliver an especially beautiful, long, lean physique—a dancer's body, even for women who had never had any dance training at all.

It wasn't long before word spread about Berk's method among dancers, actors, and Londoners in the know. In 1971, the Lotte Berk Method studio opened its doors for the first time in New York City, where the technique and its original founder quickly became a word-of-mouth success. Berk's groundbreaking synthesis of strength training, dance, and orthopedic back exercises was a brand-new combination that delivered a different kind of body and set a new standard for what the average woman could achieve through exercise. Best of all, even though the exercises were rigorous, the workouts retained a sense of femininity and fun—something few women could resist.

In the years since the Lotte Berk Method studio closed its doors, we have used the many advances in sports science and exercise physiology to further develop her technique and create a new incarnation that retains all of the fundamentals, but yields even more impressive results. The difference—and the secret that keeps us ahead of the fitness curve—lies in our own groundbreaking process: Interval Overload + Isometrics + Stretching.

How Our Formula Works

Physique 57 is an innovative form of fusion fitness that combines interval training, isometric exercises, and orthopedic stretches to systematically lengthen and sculpt your muscles to create a beautiful, sexy body. While many workouts do some form of interval training, we've taken the concept to the next level to make it even more effective. With our interval sets, your muscles are targeted and overloaded to the point of fatigue, then stretched for relief. We call this process Interval Overload. Bringing the muscle to the point of fatigue—the point where it starts to burn and shake—ensures that you are providing it with the greatest possible stimulus, and as a result you see greater changes faster, and with fewer reps. The stretches between the sets allow your muscles to recover and train them to always take their full length—so that you appear taller and more graceful, rather than muscular and bulked up.

We also make tremendous use of isometrics: exercises that challenge your muscles without any visible contractions or movements. Often, simply holding and bracing a particular muscle can be more powerful than doing a hundred reps, so we begin each of our interval sets with an isometric hold—an innovative starting position designed to engage the target muscles as well as ancillary ones before you even start doing the movements. The isometric hold not only makes the interval sets more challenging, but also pushes you to recruit additional muscles throughout the body to help you stabilize the position and perform the reps in the proper way. In this way, you end up toning far more than just the target muscle group with every single Physique 57 move.

This breakthrough process works so well because it increases your lean body mass more effectively than any other workout. Your body composition includes muscle, bone, and fat, and the percentages of each determine how you look. Two people with the exact same height and body weight can look completely different because they have different body compositions. The key, therefore, to looking slim and sexy is to not only blast away fat, but also increase your lean body mass, or muscle. You can diet all you want, but if you don't target your muscles in the right way, you're not going to see the definition that truly transforms your body. Physique 57 workouts are designed to significantly increase your lean body mass in an incredibly short amount of time. By overloading the muscles to provide them with the maximum stimulus possible and then *further* challenging them through isometrics, we are giving your muscles a one-two punch that pushes them to change at an amazingly rapid rate. We'll talk more about the science behind this process and how it works in chapter 2.

Creating lean body mass is actually harder than you'd think. For many years, strength training has been considered the most effective way to generate and build lean muscle. Lifting weights again and again not only is boring, but can also stress your joints and lead to injury over time. What's more, certain forms of exercise can actually *decrease* your lean body mass if you're not careful. If your workout focuses too heavily on cardiovascular training, for example, as with running or aerobics, you will actually *lose* lean body mass because your body breaks down muscle tissue to generate fuel (carbohydrates) for all that cardio. The same is true if you combine a heavy workout schedule with a low- or no-carb diet. In this way, you can end up sabotaging your efforts. An unintentional loss of lean body mass is one of the reasons that people can be working out frequently but still not seeing results.

The good news is that Physique 57 has been proven to deliver marked changes in lean body mass while also boosting cardiovascular health and generating significant caloric burn—a feat all the more impressive because it is done without using heavy weights or equipment. This rapid change in body composition also accounts for the dramatic loss of inches off the thighs, waist, and arms that our clients experience because, quite simply, lean muscle tissue takes up far less space than fat. The more lean body mass you have, the slimmer you will look, no matter if the numbers on the scale change very little or even remain the same.

But the advantages of better body composition don't end there: Your lean body mass also determines your resting metabolic rate (RMR), or the number of calories your body burns at rest. Increasing your lean body mass is the ONLY way to permanently boost your metabolism: Muscle tissue burns fifteen times as many calories as fat, so the more of it you have, the more calories you'll burn throughout the day, even when you're not exercising. After age thirty, a woman's RMR decreases at a rate of 2 to 3 percent per decade, so now is the time to fight back! With every Physique 57 workout, you'll be sculpting your body into a lean, mean, calorie-burning machine. And if you combine our exercise formula with our knockout eating plan, which shaves off additional calories and boosts your metabolism even more, you've got a recipe for major change, and a body capable of staying fit and slim for life.

The Physique 57 Difference

Our revolutionary combination of isometrics and Interval Overload is perhaps the most important way that we stand out from other workouts. It's the core of our process and, together with our lengthening stretches, the catalyst that boosts lean body mass and transforms your physique. But there are many other aspects of our program that are radically different from other fitness methods and contribute to the overall package and fantastic results that our clients love. Here are some of the other ways Physique 57 outshines the other techniques and regimens you've tried before.

1. **Major caloric burn.** A typical Physique 57 workout burns up to 650 calories depending on your body weight and fitness level—significantly more than other forms of exercise, including an hour of Pilates (390 calories), an hour of Spinning (300 calories), running a mile (100 calories), or even swimming a mile (400 calories). The truth is that many popular fitness methods, such as Spinning and running, actually have a surprisingly low rate of caloric burn; Spinning burns fewer calories because you are coasting on momentum for most of the workout, and running, while terrific for your cardiovascular system, just doesn't burn a lot of calories—you have to run a lot of miles to make a difference on the calorie front. And when it comes to more static exercises like yoga, forget it—you're hardly burning any calories at all!

   Physique 57's high caloric burn is a direct result of Interval Overload: Your muscles will burn more calories when you push them to the point of fatigue. When you're really feeling the burn and the heat, you've entered your optimum calorie-burning zone. Plus, our technique focuses on strengthening the muscles, and muscle tissue, as we've said, burns fifteen times as many calories as fat. The stronger you get, the more calories you'll burn during your workouts—a fabulous cycle that keeps the pounds coming off!

2. **Innovative choreography.** Our dance-inspired exercise moves are a breath of fresh air in the workout world: Instead of triceps dips, we do the Triceps Can-Can; instead of lunges, we do the Curtsy; instead of squats, we do Thigh Dancing. All of our moves are designed to be fun and feminine and to remove any sense of intimidation. With Physique 57 you can say good-bye to many dreaded moves from other workouts, including jumping jacks, jogging in place, torso twists, and endless sets of crunches.

3. **Variety.** If you walk into a class at any gym across the country, the class will

likely consist of lengthy sets of reps: eight lunges on the left side, eight on the right side, eight on the left again, and so on. It's tedious and exhausting and everyone watches the clock. In our workouts, we constantly change up the positions and the tempo, so even if you're working your thigh muscles for twenty minutes, the variety of exercises keeps you focused and challenged, and time flies by. As a bonus, working the same muscle in different ways actually builds muscle faster than doing the same moves again and again, making better results the icing on the cake.

4. **Efficiency.** Physique 57 is designed to make every second count and give you maximum results in the least amount of time. In just 57 minutes, our strategic sequence of moves works every muscle group in the body and even zeros in on different fibers within the same muscle. In addition, because of isometrics, most of our signature moves target not just one muscle group but several. In fact, we use the core muscles during 80 percent of the workout. Our Pretzel move, for example, actually works your seat muscles and your waistline so that you are simultaneously sculpting both. How's that for multitasking?

5. **It's good for you.** Despite the vigorous nature of our workouts, our moves are based on orthopedic and rehabilitative exercises, and thus provide a safe, organic way of reshaping your body. Remember, Lotte Berk originally developed her own exercise regimen as a way to strengthen and retrain her muscles after an injury. There's no pounding, as with jumping jacks or running, and our moves don't put pressure on joints and ligaments the way step aerobics or StairMasters do. Many clients who come to us with injuries say that Physique 57 is the only workout they've found that doesn't cause additional problems or pain. Our leg lifts are perfect for weak knees; strengthening your abs takes pressure off your lower back; and our weight-bearing (or standing) exercises improve bone density. You'll never finish our workouts feeling beat up. Sure, you'll feel tired, but you'll also feel energized and glowing from having challenged your body in a healthy way.

6. **It looks good, too.** If you've ever studied dance, you know that a ballet master or choreographer will often tell his dancers that their bodies should

look beautiful during every single second of a performance, and from every angle. Whether you're going into a turn or coming out of a turn, whether you're about to kick a leg up or your leg is coming down, you should always appear graceful enough that if someone snapped your picture, the photograph would turn out well. We couldn't agree more, and all of our moves and sequences have been created with this in mind. No matter how hard you're working, we want your body to look like a painting, so we've given you moves like Figure Skater, Mermaid, and Gazelle Stretch. Now, isn't that more appealing than doing sweaty, grunty squats?

While the past few years have seen an upsurge in other dance-based workouts, these regimens lack the innovative variations and sequences that Physique 57 uses to zone in on and target even your deepest muscles. Most important, they fail to challenge your muscles to the point of overload—and unless you hit that sweet spot where you're really feeling the heat, you're not going to see the truly transformative changes you desire.

The Anatomy of a Physique 57 Workout

A Physique 57 workout is designed to target and tone every muscle group in the body in just 57 minutes. The six different series within the workout—Warm-Up, Thighs, Seat, Abs, Back, and Cool Down—comprise anywhere from one to three sections. Each section is made up of moves, and each move consists of different sets of reps called variations. Together the moves and variations build on one another to systematically sculpt every one of your muscles and ensure that you remain in the calorie-burning zone. We also stretch in between sections to release and lengthen the muscles you've been working, and give your body a chance to recharge so that you can start the next section even stronger.

Because we know boredom saps both strength and enthusiasm, we've structured the workout so that no one section within a series ever takes longer than eight minutes, and many take far less. You won't believe how easy it is to get through a killer thigh sequence when you know you only have three minutes to go before you stretch. And within the sections themselves, we rarely spend longer than a minute working the muscles in any given position. This rapid-fire pacing keeps you present and focused on the moves and variations you're performing so that you can really give it your all with every rep.

The six different series within the workout are:

1. Warm-Up (8 minutes)

A Physique 57 warm-up is unlike any other. We don't devote time to stretches or gentle aerobics—instead, we grab our free weights and dive right in. While biceps curls and push-ups might be the main event in other workouts, for us they're just the beginning. Our warm-ups will get your heart rate up and start the caloric burn; plus, this is where we do some of our best shoulder- and arm-sculpting work. Most people don't realize that working your arm muscles burns the *least* amount of calories of any muscle group in your body, so we do our main push for the arms here rather than giving them a separate series of their own. We use free weights to generate heat and sculpt your biceps, triceps, and shoulders in a very short amount of time.

2. Thighs (15 minutes)

The thighs are the largest muscle group in your body, and they generate the biggest calorie burn; thus, we spend a lot of our time working them because they are your single best ally in reshaping your body. Our Thigh series is split into three different sections, each followed by accompanying stretches; because the muscles themselves are so large, you really need a variety of moves to hit all the trouble spots. The first two sections are done standing up and use different leg positions to target your thighs from every angle, as well as the lower leg muscles, especially the calves. The third section is always Thigh Dancing, one of our signature moves that gets you down on the floor and provides a fun, ultra-efficient way to sculpt your quads *and* waistline. Together these moves are guaranteed to shrink-wrap your thighs, smoothing and slimming them to be fabulously jiggle-free. Just watch those inches disappear!

3. Seat (14 minutes)

Almost every workout regimen targets the gluteus maximus—the two large muscles that form the curve of your buttocks and determine whether you have a shapely, lifted seat. But the seat area also includes the gluteus medius, minimus, and dozens of other tiny muscles that are equally important if you want to look great in your sexy undies or bikini bottoms. In this third series, we work all the angles of the seat to make sure that we're hitting every single one of those muscles, with a focus on the lower seat, which is where we store the most fat. The first half of our seat work is done standing up to give you a healthy dose of isometrics as you work to maintain the proper postures; the second half is done on the floor, which enables you to go deeper and target the glutes' innermost muscle fibers. As always, we stretch when we finish each side to release those seat muscles, relieve the burn, and get you fired up and ready for more!

4. Abs (14 minutes)

Our totally unique abdominal series includes three sets of moves done in three different positions: Flat Back, Round Back, and Curl. These moves and their variations are incredibly effective at involving and strengthening all four sets of abdominal muscles: the rectus abdominis, the transversus abdominis, and the internal and external obliques. Each position changes the angle of the spine to give you a new isometric hold, which in turn enables you to recruit and engage different muscles. As a result, you can sculpt and cinch even the deepest layers of the entire abdominal wall—something that traditional sit-ups and crunches fail to do. Because we know that ab work is agony for many people, we only spend three to four minutes in each of the positions and intersperse fun moves like the Forearm Plank and Triceps Dips. And rather than stretching between each section, we hold the stretches for your abs until we've finished working the other side of your core, the back. We keep things moving so that before you know it, it's over—and yet you've hit those abdominals harder than you ever have before!

5. Back (3 minutes)

Often we spend so much time focusing on how our front looks that we forget about the other side altogether. But strong and supple back muscles are an essential part of our trademark physique, and we spend time on these muscles, even if most workouts don't. This series complements the upper back work already done in our Warm-Up by focusing on the middle and lower back. We start off with Back Dancing, a sexy way of strengthening the lower back that also hits the glutes one more time, and follow that with Back Extensors—a quick sequence of moves that engage your lower back, middle back, and core, and help create flexibility in the spine. This series leads to better posture, making you look taller and more graceful.

6. Cool Down (3 minutes)

Ahhhh…at last! In these last few minutes of the workout, we move through a series of stretches to relax and elongate your tired muscles, and bring your heart rate back to normal. Since you've already been stretching throughout, there's no need for anything more elaborate. A few last moves and you're ready to go, stronger, healthier, and energized from knowing that you were brave enough to challenge yourself—and you won!

The Props: How We Enhance Your Workouts

At Physique 57, we believe that your own body is and always should be your very best workout tool. After all, exercise should prepare you to move with strength and assuredness through daily life, and we don't go about our days with weights strapped to our wrists or a Nautilus machine draped over our shoulders. Therefore, the majority of our workout moves require nothing more than your own muscles and determination. If you do the moves correctly while maintaining the proper form, and push yourself to increase your precision and stamina, you're going to see big changes as a result.

That said, there are several props we employ during our workouts to help you get the most out of the moves and ensure that you achieve Interval Overload. Several of these props, such as a chair and cushion, are used to help you find and maintain the proper position throughout the movements. This is especially important when you're first starting the workout and your muscles are not yet strong enough to hold you in place without support. Others, such as free weights and playground balls, are used to create additional resistance and help you recruit more muscle than you could if you were doing the same movements on your own. Here's the skinny on the props that you will be using and how they facilitate and enhance your workouts:

- **A chair or sturdy piece of furniture.** When we teach classes at our studios, we use a ballet barre for support—this, of course, being the traditional tool used by dancers to help them build strength and balance. For your at-home routine, we suggest that you hold on to the back of a chair or a sturdy, waist-high piece of furniture. Used during the Thigh and Seat series, the chair serves the exact same purpose as the barre, and will help you find and maintain the proper position for each movement. It will also give you some additional support in the beginning while you're learning the moves and strengthening the muscles that will help you maintain each move's isometric hold.

- **A two- to three-inch-thick cushion.** In the Curl section of our Ab series, the cushion serves the exact same purpose as the chair, helping you maintain the proper form and position—and in particular keep a neutral spine, which is essential for effective, injury-free ab work. *Neutral spine* refers to the natural curve of your lower back. By placing a cushion on the floor directly behind you, you prevent excessive arching in this area and force the lower abdominals to engage and hold the spine in place. Plus, it provides some extra padding for your middle back, or thoracic spine, as you curl up and down off the floor. If you don't have access to a cushion of this size, you can use a folded towel (or towels) instead.

- **A playground ball.** We use the playground ball throughout our workouts to increase the intensity of certain moves in a playful way, and also to help isolate and target critical yet hard-to-work muscles such as the adductors, or inner thighs. Your adductors don't get a lot of everyday use, so placing and squeezing the ball between your thighs concentrates the movement on those muscles in a way that is difficult to do with only your body's own weight as resistance. We also use the ball as a source of support and stability for some of our floor work.

■ **Free weights.** While your body is the sole machinery for most of our workout moves, we do use free weights during our Warm-Up to further challenge the arm, upper back, and shoulder muscles. Although we also target these muscles through Push-Ups, Triceps Dips, and other moves that use the body's own weight as resistance, our standing upper body moves require additional resistance to bring the muscles to the point of overload. Our Warm-Up uses two different sets of handheld weights: a lighter set of three to five pounds, and a heavier set of five to eight pounds, depending on your fitness level. As a rule, we like using heavier weights because they produce bigger changes with fewer reps; we can sculpt the arm muscles quickly and efficiently, and then move on.

How to Use This Book

The premise of our two-week plan is simple: Do our workouts five times a week and follow our suggested meal plans and you will achieve the body you've always wanted. The two 57-minute workouts presented in part 3 are designed to work together and target your muscles in different ways, so you should alternate between them for a total of at least five workouts a week. If you're already in pretty good shape and want to do more, go for it! Just be sure that you always switch off between the workouts to get the maximum benefit and variety of moves. But no matter how fit you are, we recommend at least one "free" day per week to give your muscles a chance to recover and recharge.

Although it may be tempting to dive right in, we strongly encourage you to take some time before starting the program to familiarize yourself with the steps for each of the moves in part 2. Your workouts will be far more effective if you don't have to pause to flip back through the book for more detailed instructions; ideally you want to be comfortable enough with each move that you can see the name, a photo, and the number of reps, and be ready to go. In part 2, we'll provide more specific guidance on practicing the moves and preparing for your workouts, but in the meantime keep in mind that practice reps DO count—you're still moving your body, working your muscles, and training them to help you get the most out of your efforts.

We also recommend spacing out your free days each week rather than taking them back-to-back. When you're first starting the program, try to resist the urge to take a day off right at the very beginning, even if you're sore (and you probably will be!). Soreness is a GOOD thing. It means your muscles are starting to change, and contrary to what some people believe, working out with sore muscles isn't harmful—in fact, keeping those muscles loose and limber will help the soreness disappear more quickly. So at the outset, try to do the workouts at least three days in a row before taking a break—you want to build momentum and keep it going!

When it comes to the meal plan, advance preparation is your ally here as well. Part 4 explains our philosophy of healthy eating and provides quick-and-easy steps for a Kitchen Makeover, two weeks' worth of shopping lists, and Girl-on-the-Go suggestions for eating out that you can use to fit your lifestyle—all of which you should use to prepare yourself and your pantry for the weeks ahead. We then provide meal plans and recipes for each of the fourteen days, including breakfasts, lunches, dinners, and snacks. We recommend that you start the plan on a Monday, which gives you the weekend to shop and prepare some dishes in advance, particularly the various dressings and sauces that can be used in a number of ways. Taking the time to eliminate some of the prep work will make it far easier to stick with the meal plan once Monday arrives and your busy life resumes. As you continue on the program, you can use your free days off from working out to pick up additional groceries and plan for upcoming meals.

We'd also like to suggest that for these two weeks, you put your late-night social life on hold and prioritize getting a good night's sleep. We know that it's hard to resist a cocktail or two, but your body is going to be working harder than it has in a while, and getting enough rest will ensure that you can attack your workouts with optimum energy and vigor. The healthier you are over the course of the program—and this includes sleeping well in addition to following our guidelines for healthy eating—the more support you will be giving your body and the more dramatic the end results will be.

HOW TO DO THE PROGRAM: A SAMPLE TWO-WEEK SCHEDULE

Starting the program on a Monday is the easiest option for many people, and the one that we feel best sets you up for success. If you do choose to start on a Monday, here is how your schedule might look:

Week 1

Monday: Day 1, Workout A

Tuesday: Day 2, Workout B

Wednesday: Day 3, Workout A

Thursday: Day 4, Free Day

Friday: Day 5, Workout B

Saturday: Day 6, Workout A

Sunday: Day 7, Free Day

Week 2

Monday: Day 8, Workout B

Tuesday: Day 9, Workout A

Wednesday: Day 10, Free Day

Thursday: Day 11, Workout B

Friday: Day 12, Workout A

Saturday: Day 13, Workout B

Sunday: Day 14, Free Day

We hope that you will fall in love with Physique 57 and want to continue doing the workouts and enjoying our healthy recipes even after these first two weeks are up. And the good news is that you can, because your body will only get better and better! We still strive to perfect the moves ourselves, to work a little harder, to go a little deeper, and to keep feeling the burn, even though we've been practicing the technique for years. And we can tell you honestly that the rewards and the challenges never stop.

You'll feel amazing when you finish the program in this book—but right now, you should revel in the fun of getting started and get psyched about the incredible transformation that lies ahead. You're just fourteen days away from looking strong, slim, and sexy. Let's go!

2

SCIENCE CAN MAKE YOU SEXY

WITH SO MANY DIETS AND FITNESS PLANS TO CHOOSE from, it can be tough to tell what's hype and what's not. Today it often seems like every personal trainer is hawking a brand-new method to help you get in shape and lose weight faster than ever before: "In just ten days!" ... "In just six sessions!" ... "In just eight minutes, three mornings a week!" Most of us hear these promises and know deep down they CAN'T be true. But that doesn't stop us from trying them anyway, hoping that this time the program is for real and we've finally found the secret to looking great for life.

At first glance, Physique 57 might seem like just another pie-in-the-sky miracle workout. After all, a loss of ten inches and ten pounds in just two weeks is pretty extraordinary! But we're here to tell you that our program is firmly grounded in the established, proven principles of science and exercise physiology, and that's how we deliver on the amazing results we promise. And as we mentioned, our workouts are also founded on principles of orthopedic and rehabilitative exercise, which is why, even as challenging as they are, they are so incredibly healthy for your bones, joints, muscles, and mind. Everything that we promise IS possible because it all falls within the parameters of what your body is designed to do—our workouts fire up your body's own natural strengthening and weight-loss mechanisms, kick them into high gear, and ultimately supercharge them so they become more powerful and efficient than ever before.

This chapter offers a closer look at the science behind our technique, particularly the physiology involved in our process of Interval Overload. It also explores exactly how the different workout components fit together to produce our signature long, lean physique. When you know that our promises are backed by science, you will also KNOW that the Physique 57 transformation is truly within your grasp. And that's the very best kind of motivation you can have!

So now it's time to set aside any lingering doubts about whether or not our program can work for you. We're going to give you the inside scoop on our innovative method, and delve into the details of how our program works, and why.

The Science of Interval Overload

Interval training has been widely recognized for years as an extremely effective form of exercise. Bursts of high-intensity work are alternated with periods of lower-intensity activity or rest. The idea is that by taking these breaks, you are able to increase your overall output: The brief recovery periods allow you to work harder during the high-intensity periods and continue to exercise for a longer amount of time. Numerous studies have shown that interval training truly does deliver the goods: It is incredibly efficient not only at improving your cardiovascular health and stamina—it increases the body's aerobic capacity to exercise longer at varying intensities—but also at creating lean body mass, that all-important body component that determines how you look. As we discussed in chapter 1, increasing your lean body mass also boosts your metabolism and rate of caloric burn, making interval training one of the most effective ways to spark fat loss as well. It is the preferred mode of training among athletes, and with good reason: The results are consistent and quantifiable, far surpassing any that can be achieved through simply doing an hour of activity—whether jogging or yoga—at a constant pace.

Physique 57's interval training regimen is designed to amplify both the process and the results. We stretch between sets to lengthen the muscles and allow them to recharge so that you can start your next section even stronger. But stretching isn't the only thing we do during our recoveries; often, we'll shift the focus and work a different set of muscles. For example, we'll do thirty seconds of Triceps Dips in between our first and second Ab sections, which gives your abs a chance to recover while simultaneously activating and sculpting the arms. Even within the same set, we will often switch from working one muscle to another (for example, from inner thighs to quads, then back to inner thighs), or between different parts of the same muscle. In this way, you get all the benefits of interval training, while also continuing to work different muscles during your recovery so you can make the most of every minute and keep the caloric burn going.

Our interval training sets are designed not only to challenge the muscles, but also to give them the MAXIMUM STIMULUS POSSIBLE. We do this not just by working them hard—after all, that's what most workouts do—but by pushing them all the way to overload, or to the point known in exercise physiology as momentary muscular fatigue. And when you reach that point—when your muscles are burning and shaking, and can no longer contract even if you try—you know that you've also reached the absolute peak of your intensity. You've activated those muscles as much as you possibly can, and you'll absolutely need to take a break if you want them to perform any more.

Achieving overload may not feel fabulous in the moment, but you *should* feel great about it, because it's when you hit that point that three major physiological changes take place. First, by stimulating the muscle to such a tremendous degree, you've activated the neural pathways between your brain and that muscle at a very high level. These pathways are how your brain sends signals to your muscles to tell them to contract, and by activating these pathways again and again at a high intensity, you create a baseline of activation in the muscle. This means that your muscle fibers remain partially activated, or contracted (as opposed to limp and flaccid) at *all* times, and this accounts for what we call firmness, or tone. The greater your baseline of activation, the firmer your muscles will be. And that's what makes the jiggle disappear!

Second, stimulating these neural pathways also allows you to recruit more individual muscle fibers within any given muscle, and this is what determines strength.

Whenever you use a muscle—whether you're lifting or standing or walking down the street—you have the opportunity to activate anywhere from 5 percent to 100 percent of the muscle fibers, depending on your level of conditioning. The more your brain keeps firing signals along those neural pathways, the greater the number of muscle fibers that will respond. You ultimately become stronger because you're building new neural pathways that are more efficient than ever before, and using more fibers within each muscle as a result. Even better, the more muscle fibers you use, the more calories you'll burn during your workouts. This is one of the reasons that most Physique 57 clients drop pounds without even having to diet.

The third major change that takes place occurs on a cellular level within the actual fibers themselves. Contrary to popular belief, you cannot actually "build" new muscle fibers—you are born with a set number of fibers in each muscle that is largely determined by genetics. But you CAN build more strands of actin and myosin, the protein filaments within each fiber that are responsible for moving your muscles, thus increasing your muscles' strength and power, and changing their size and shape, which is what gives you definition. Bringing a muscle to the point of overload will push it to grow actin and myosin faster than regular interval training or any other form of exercise. When the muscle reaches the point of momentary muscular fatigue, it knows it has to adapt to the stimulus being provided, so it responds by growing new strands of these all-important proteins so that it will be ready the next time. Once again, these changes result in greater caloric burn—stronger muscle fibers use more energy, and the more energy you need, the more likely it is that your body will start breaking down fat to fuel the movements.

Of course, the key to Physique 57's Interval Overload is that there is no time at which your muscles are perfectly adapted and able to breeze through our sets with ease. No matter how fit or familiar with the program you are, we ALWAYS take you to the point of overload. We keep changing the pace, the moves, and the angles to make sure that you always feel the burn and reach that sweet spot where transformation is taking place. We hit these same muscles again and again, sculpting and toning them to give you a lean, gorgeous shape and a rock-star metabolism that will keep you thin for life. But Interval Overload is far from the only way that Physique 57 stimulates change in your muscles. Even as you're fighting your way through sets of reps, we're working your muscles in a second way that many consider to be equally challenging: isometrics.

The Beauty of Isometrics

When it comes to fitness, there are only two kinds of exercises you can do: isotonic and isometric. Isotonic, or dynamic, exercises are what we usually envision when we think about working out. These are the exercises that make you move: Your muscles contract, your joints bend, and your limbs shift from one position to another. Most important, the length of the muscle changes as it contracts through a *range of motion*. When you do a biceps curl, for example, your biceps muscle starts out longer and shortens bit by bit until you achieve a full contraction. The reps, or variations, that we do in our interval sets to bring you to the point of overload are isotonics: From hip shakes to curl-ups to squeezes on the ball, all of these exercises have you moving your body and stimulating your muscles as a result.

Isometric exercises, on the other hand, stimulate the muscles without any visible contractions or movements. With isometrics, you contract and then *brace* your muscles to hold the body in a static position, rather than move through a range of motion. The muscle is engaged, but there is no movement as there is with isotonics. Instead, you find the optimum point in the contraction and stay there. Yoga, for example, is highly isometric—there are subtle movements that take you from position to position, but mainly you're finding and then holding the postures. Isometrics are also at work when you keep your abs pulled in and your spine aligned during push-ups, or hold your arm above your head during barre work in ballet.

If you think that isometrics sound easy compared with isotonics, trust us—they're not! If you've ever tried to hold a Roman Chair position against a wall for more than a minute or two, you know that isometrics can be TOUGH. In fact, often simply holding and bracing a particular muscle can be just as rigorous as targeting it through reps because you're not relying on momentum from the movement to carry you through. You can even achieve overload through isometrics if the muscle contraction is challenging enough and you hold it for an ample amount of time. Even a move as basic as holding a playground ball over your head can really fire up the muscles in your arms, shoulders, and core.

There are two significant advantages to performing isometrics: The first is that they tend to activate a lot of smaller, ancillary muscles that get overlooked if you focus solely on isotonics. Isotonic movements, by their nature, tend to work just one or two muscles at a time—and while that can be very effective, it's also limiting. You can't, for example, spot-target every single one of the tiny muscles in your seat or every inch of the inner abdominal wall through isotonic movements. The muscles are simply too small and too deep. However, engaging a larger area of the body in an isometric hold can actually recruit and stimulate those hidden muscles as they are called upon to keep you stable and help the larger muscles maintain the position. Holding your torso at a forty-five-degree incline, for example, during your thigh work, engages the entire core in a way that doing a simple curl-up will not. Similarly, maintaining a T position with your upper body during seat work (see our Figure Skater move, page 94) will not only activate your back and core, but also increase the intensity on the glutes and surrounding seat muscles. Ultimately, isometrics are a fantastic way to involve more muscles, especially hard-to-reach ones, in every move.

We also love these subtle yet potent exercises because they tone your muscles without increasing their size, ensuring that you retain a slender, feminine shape. On a cellular level, isometrics produce many of the same changes as isotonics: They stimulate the neural pathways in your muscle fibers to produce a greater baseline of activity, which in turn leads to greater strength, firmness, and tone. However, because you are bracing and holding the muscles in place rather than moving them through a range of motion, the changes you see in the shape of the muscle are less pronounced. In this way, isometrics are an essential part of what creates our signature long, lithe, dancer's physique: They tone the muscles but avoid adding bulk.

As we discussed in chapter 1, isometrics provide the foundation for almost every one of our workout moves. Each move begins with an isometric hold, or starting position, that is specifically designed to fire up your ancillary muscles and make the interval sets or reps for that move more challenging and effective. For example, in Standing Crane (page 91), you begin by standing with both hands on your chair, your torso angled slightly forward, and your right leg bent to bring the right heel up behind your seat muscle. From there, you go on to perform your reps—pulses, knee circles, and other isotonic movements designed to get you to Interval Overload—all while keeping the working leg bent at the proper angle and maintaining the position of the torso. The isotonic reps target the glutes, so that's where you're going to feel the burn. But with the isometric hold, you're also activating your hamstrings, calves, core, and even upper arms.

Isometrics are certainly at the heart of our workouts, and you'll even find that the names of the moves themselves—Power Plié, Skier, Curtsy, Clam, and so on—are specifically designed to cue these all-important starting positions and remind you of where you need to be before beginning your reps. But it's the reps themselves that give each of these moves their "movement." So let's take a closer look at what makes up our interval sets: a sequence of moves *within* each move called the variations.

The Variations

When it comes to exercise, we believe that variety is the secret to keeping people motivated and engaged during a workout. Luckily, it's also one of the very best ways to tone and strengthen muscles. Whereas most interval training sets involve performing the same activity again and again, our interval sets are built around a sequence of *different* movements, or what we call variations. You're still working the same muscle or muscle group, and the isometric hold, or starting position, remains unchanged. But when it comes to the actual reps, we vary the choreography so that in most instances, you'll never perform the same kind of movement or rep more than sixteen times in a row.

The variations are what give each move that all-important *range of motion* that stimulates muscle change and leads to Interval Overload. For example, from our Small V starting position, we go on to perform five different variations: Pulses, Hip Tucks, Hip Shakes, Hip Circles, and Deep Pliés, or knee bends that lower your seat toward the floor. Together these variations encompass a greater range of movement and work the thigh and seat muscles more thoroughly than any single one could on its own—even if you performed it a hundred times. And that's the best part: When we string them together, we only need to perform each variation for thirty to sixty seconds at a time to get the maximum benefit—and thirty to sixty seconds is nothing! But make no mistake, the effect is cumulative: By the time you reach the end of a set, your muscles WILL be burning and shaking. You've achieved overload, but you've done it in a way that *feels* far easier than doing three straight minutes of Hip Circles.

Variations are a large part of what enables us to target all of your muscles and give them the maximum stimulus possible in such a short amount of time. With each new variation, we change the height of your leg, the position of your feet, or the direction of the movement in order to stimulate and sculpt the muscles in different ways. Sometimes just shifting by a matter of inches enables you to target a whole new set of muscle fibers. As a result, Physique 57 involves more planes and ranges of motion than any other workout, even Pilates, making it comparable only to dance. Changing the angles and movement patterns also helps to prevent the kind of stress injuries that can result from working the same muscles and joints again and again in the same way. We also include a good number of standing, or weight-bearing, variations because these help to improve bone density—especially important for women as we get older.

These variations are also another major reason that our clients rarely, if ever, plateau. People often reach exercise plateaus because they become bored with what they're doing and stop challenging themselves. But our workouts move so quickly and contain such a variety of activity that our clients remain excited to take them on. There are literally hundreds of ways to put together a Physique 57 workout, two of which are featured in this book. Plus, facing a new challenge every thirty to sixty seconds will inspire you to perfect every one of the variations, to do them better and more fluidly as you keep up with the tempo. And if you get tired or find one of the variations especially challenging, you needn't worry—there's a new one right around the corner, and you can dive back in and attack the next set of reps with renewed vigor. As a bonus, this rapid-fire pacing gives our workout a healthy dose of cardio: Performing ten Push-Ups in thirty seconds and then moving on definitely gets your heart rate up, as will the variations that involve multiple muscle groups.

Our interval sets generally comprise two to three moves, each of which includes anywhere from two to ten variations. If that sounds like a lot, remember that each variation only takes thirty to sixty seconds to perform—so a single Thigh section may only take three to four minutes. Still, we pack A LOT of effort into those four minutes! And with your muscles getting such an incredible amount of stimulus from all these variations, isometrics, and Interval Overload, the rate of body transformation can be rapid and dramatic. That is why throughout our interval sets, we don't stop simply to rest, but to *stretch* and lengthen your muscles at every turn.

The Stretches

Anytime you stimulate a muscle through exercise, you're doing so in order to provoke change. By stimulating the muscle again and again, you're attempting to rewire its neural pathways to keep it in a moderate state of contraction, or activation—to achieve that baseline of neural activity that we previously discussed—rather than simply letting it hang there, limp and flaccid.

It is at this point that stretching, the third key element that defines a Physique 57 workout, comes into play. Stretching between our interval sets allows us to reclaim the full length of our muscles while still maintaining the new baseline of activation that we've achieved. We believe that stretching throughout your workout rather than waiting until the end is one of the secrets to producing a long, lean shape; stretching your thighs immediately after performing a vigorous Thigh series, for example, not only provides a welcome release for those muscles, but also trains them to always take their full length. In addition, your muscles respond best to stretching when they're warm, so stretching immediately after the series, right after you've generated all that heat, allows you to go as deep as possible into the stretch, lengthening and smoothing the muscles without risking an injury or tear. We don't spend a lot of time on these stretches as a rule—just twenty to thirty seconds apiece—because we don't want to derail the momentum of your workout. We want to keep you in the calorie-burning zone and keep your heart rate up, so we move through them quickly, and then get right back to the next section.

Some of our clients initially wonder if doing these brief stretches interspersed throughout the workout is as effective or advantageous as stretching for longer periods of time. After all, in the past, most workout DVDs and fitness classes have started and ended with five to ten minutes of stretching. But in recent years, several major studies have shown that a lengthy stretching period isn't all it's cracked up to be. These studies concluded that the maximum benefit you can get from any stretch is achieved somewhere in the range of fifteen to thirty seconds. Holding a stretch for two minutes or more won't get you any further than stretching for twenty seconds. Similarly, they found that repeating a stretch ten times in one workout gives you no greater benefit than simply doing it once. Physique 57 strives for optimum benefits and efficiency, so we do each stretch once, for twenty to thirty seconds, when each particular muscle group is warmed and most receptive. In this way, our toned and firm muscles become long, supple, and flexible as well, and we get that all-important recovery part of the interval process. Many of our clients tell us that if they *don't* stretch between sets, they feel less limber throughout the workout and can't give each section their all as a result.

Stretching also has real orthopedic benefits, helping to protect you from strain and injury. Tighter muscles that cannot easily take their full length may put pressure on joints and tear more readily, whether you're hiking in the mountains, carrying heavy packages, or just moving about in the course of your everyday life. So if you're tempted to skip the stretches in our workouts, remember that you're not just stretching to achieve lithe, gorgeous muscles—you're also stretching to maintain a healthy body.

How It All Comes Together

In chapter 1, we explored the structure of a Physique 57 workout and saw how the six different series fit together: Warm-Up, Thighs, Seat, Abs, Back, and Cool Down. But within each of these series, the moves themselves follow a deliberate and precise sequence that is designed to engage every single one of your muscles, prevent injury, and help you achieve Interval Overload as quickly as possible. The order of the moves and the timing in each section work together for maximum efficiency—we give you exactly what you need, no more and no less, to achieve your optimum results. Everything you need to get a great body is contained in our 57-minute workout. It's going to be challenging, but as our clients like to say, "It's the hardest hour you'll ever love!"

And you're not going to have to do it alone—we'll be with you every step of the way. We'll help you find the rhythm by counting the reps and giving you upbeat music that makes you want to move. You'll be surprised at how natural the movements will start to feel after just a few sessions, and before long you'll be amazed at what your body can actually do. The isometric holds will become second nature, you'll breeze through the variations with confidence, and you'll love the feeling you get when you realize you CAN go the distance and fight through the burn to finish the sets. Even from one workout to the next, you are going to feel your muscles getting stronger and see changes in tone and definition that let you know, THIS IS WORKING! And there's no motivator like success.

So now that you know how the program works, let's get right to part 2 and start learning the moves. It's time to create some long, lean muscles! Let the transformation begin.

PART TWO

THE MOVES

AT LAST, IT'S TIME TO START LEARNING THE MOVES THAT
will appear in your workouts for the next two weeks. In this section of the book,
we provide step-by-step instructions for each of our exercises—the starting positions, the variations, and the accompanying stretches—and give you everything
you need to take on your first Physique 57 workout, including modifications for
beginners, advanced variations for the more adventurous, and plenty of coaching
and motivational tips to keep you inspired and fired up.

As we said in chapter 1, we highly recommend that you practice and familiarize yourself with these moves before attempting to do the workouts. While some
of them—such as Push-Ups, Biceps Curls, or Triceps Dips—may initially seem familiar, we've put a unique, Physique 57 spin on every exercise, so taking the time
to read through and practice the steps will give you a huge advantage going
forward. In general, the descriptions are broken into two parts: the Setup, which
provides instructions for the starting position, or isometric hold; and the Variations,
which outlines the steps for performing each of the variations along with notes

about form, pacing, and flow to help you put it all together and get the most out of every move. Each exercise also includes photographs to help you find the proper positioning and range of movement. Remember, with Physique 57, the magic is in the details, so a matter of only a few inches in your positioning can make a big difference in how many inches you lose overall.

We also recommend that you wear comfortable, formfitting clothes to do your workouts. You want to be able to see the muscles you are working and accurately assess your posture and alignment, and you can't do either of these things if you're wearing sweats and a baggy T-shirt. Yoga pants—either full-length or capri—are an ideal choice because keeping your legs covered will also help you keep the heat in your thighs and hamstrings. Similarly, we recommend that your shirt or tank top cover your waist so that you can maintain as much heat in your abs as possible. And most important, no shoes! Doing our workouts barefoot gives you better stability and allows you to be more precise with your foot positions. You will also engage more ancillary leg muscles, especially in the calves and lower leg—another bonus.

Practicing the Variations: The Importance of Micromovements

When it comes to practicing the variations, there are a few that you will spot again and again throughout the six different series of the workout: pulses, tucks, circles, and microbends. These are small and simple, yet highly effective movements that can be used to sculpt a variety of muscle groups with a laser-like precision. We love these variations because their smaller range of movement is like a chisel that allows you to get deeper into the muscle. Plus, they provide a nice interlude between the larger, cardio-inducing movements that can leave you momentarily winded. But make no mistake—these moves prove that it's not the size but the intensity that counts. You WILL feel all of these "micromovements," even if at first glance they seem fairly basic:

- **Pulses.** A pulse is a small, controlled movement in which we either lift or lower a given part of the body over a very short range of motion—only about two or three inches. We do pulses for thighs, the seat, and even the back, and we like them because they provide a kind of middle ground between isometrics and some of the larger, more sweeping isotonic movements. We'll often use them to start off a new series of moves, as pulsing is a good way to get settled in a new starting position and get the burn going without diving into a full range of movement right away. We also return to pulses in between sets of more challenging reps because they give you a bit of a break and a chance to recheck your alignment, but keep the energy and caloric burn going since you're not coming to a complete stop. In fact, we'll often tell our clients that if they ever need to take a break from one of the larger movements, they can pulse for thirty seconds and then jump back in.

- **Tucks**. Hip Tucks are small, deliberate movements in which you roll your hips forward and then release them back. We perform them in the Thigh and Back series of our workout. We love this variation because no matter which muscle group you're working, Hip Tucks bring your abs and glutes into the mix and zero in on the area right below your navel (the so-called kangaroo pouch that every woman wants to avoid). We like to tell our clients, "Every time you tuck, you're giving yourself a tuck!" These small, controlled movements also strengthen the pelvic floor muscles and loosen up your lower back. Plus, they're a little bit sexy and just plain fun!

- **Circles**. Throughout our Thigh and Seat series, we regularly use our hips, legs, knees, or feet to draw small circles in the air while the rest of the body maintains an isometric hold. These tiny circles help you to engage the ancillary muscles that support the thighs and gluteal muscles. We like to think of our circles as a way to "connect the dots"—you're connecting everything together, target muscles and ancillary ones, working them in unison and toning and sculpting both as you trace the path of the circle with precision and control. You can almost see your muscles becoming tighter and more defined before your eyes!

- **Microbends**. A microbend is a deep, super-focused movement that involves bending and then straightening the leg in a very small, controlled way. The bend is slight, only a matter of inches, but it still delivers a tremendous challenge to the leg muscles because they have to work hard to control the range of movement. When you straighten the leg, you are pressing out, extending the muscles to produce a longer, straighter leg. Microbends are designed to elicit that truly full extension—something that doesn't occur naturally in most workout moves.

As you read through the exercises in the chapters that follow, you'll spot these and other components of our technique: the isometric holds, the graceful dance-based movements, and the stretches that will give you a lean and feminine shape. This is where it all starts to come together, and micromovements are just one part of the big picture. If it initially seems like there's a lot to master in these pages, don't worry. Our moves all have an inherent logic that makes performing them a lot easier than you'd think. Just take your time, be patient with yourself, and recognize that there is a learning curve.

If you're already in good shape and tempted to do more—for example, some additional moves to tighten your least favorite trouble spots—each of the chapters provides a list of Booster moves that you can use to supplement your workouts. You can tack these moves on to the end of your workout or do them when you have a few extra minutes during the day. But you don't *need* to do them—everything you need to get a great body is contained in the two classic workouts in part 3.

So now let's get acquainted with the very first moves you'll encounter anytime you cue up your playlist and begin a Physique 57 workout: the eight-minute, heat-producing series known as our Warm-Up.

A Note on Breathing

No matter how you exercise, proper breathing is essential. Not only does it enhance the cardio aspect of your workout, but it also ensures that your muscles have ample oxygen, thus improving your power and stability, and enabling you to perform at a higher level. You ideally want to breathe in rhythm with your body's movements: Whenever possible, try to *exhale* during the muscle contraction and *inhale* when the muscle relaxes or lengthens. Especially when you are doing abdominal work, you want to exhale every time you curl up to contract your abs deeper and tighter. The most important thing, however, is to KEEP BREATHING at a steady pace, even when you're concentrating or working hard to maintain a position. Holding your breath while exercising can lead to dizziness and fatigue, which can undermine your efforts. And nobody wants that!

3

WARM-UP

FOR MANY YEARS, THE WARM-UP HAS BEEN CONSIDERED the "easy" part of any fitness regimen—a mild prelude that knocks five minutes off your workout before you take on the more challenging routines. But most Physique 57 clients will agree that our warm-up is unlike any other. We don't believe in wasting your time with light aerobics or gentle stretching; instead, we want to get your muscles fired up and start generating some serious heat! So we skip the slow build and dive right in, using our free weights to get your muscles pumping, your heart rate up, and your metabolism stoked so that your body is primed for peak performance and will remain that way throughout your workout. We often hear new clients say, "That's the *warm-up*?" after they finish their first series because our starting moves are just as intense as the main moves in other workouts. But that's what makes our warm-up so effective, and why it paves the way for your success going forward.

The purpose of the warm-up has always been to set the stage for optimum results. If you want to create significant changes within your muscles, you need to create the proper conditions for change to occur—and we do this by literally warming the body. Anytime you activate a muscle, you generate heat as a by-product of the movement. And when you generate heat, a host of positive changes take place on a cellular level that make it easier for your muscles to perform at a high intensity. First, your body begins redirecting blood flow, sending more blood to the muscles that are working. Second, the heat boosts your body's oxygen dissociation curve—the rate at which your red blood cells unload and deliver oxygen to your muscles. Third, heat speeds up the all-important enzymes that control your metabolic process, causing you to start burning more calories. Whenever we do a Physique 57 Warm-Up, we like to talk about "launching into the calorie-burning zone." Ultimately, the more heat you get going in your body, the better your muscles will perform and the more calories you'll burn along the way, all of which paves the way for you to see greater changes down the line.

As you move through our Warm-Up, you will also discover that we steer clear of the usual moves like jumping jacks, side bends, step-touches, and torso twists. While we do include some classic moves such as planks, biceps curls, and triceps dips, we've either modified them to make them more interesting, or slightly changed the pace and choreography to amp them up and make them super-challenging.

For us, the Warm-Up is also the time when we do some of our best shoulder- and arm-sculpting work. Because your arm and shoulder muscles make up one of the body's smaller muscle groups, they burn far fewer calories per minute of activity than, for example, the thighs. So as we mentioned earlier, rather than giving them a separate series of their own, we fold them in here and use free weights to generate heat and provide them with the maximum stimulus possible in a very short amount of time. The arm-sculpting part of the Warm-Up takes just under five minutes and tones your biceps, triceps, pecs, shoulder, and upper back muscles to deliver a slim and sexy upper body that will have you looking gorgeous in tank tops and strapless dresses—amazing when you consider that many fitness regimens spend ten to fifteen minutes on arms alone!

When it comes to choosing and working with weights, we strongly feel that heavier is better. Contrary to what many women believe, using heavier weights will NOT cause you to bulk up—in fact, heavier weights will allow you to perform fewer reps and see better results. We recommend that you use two different sets of weights to do your Warm-Up: a lighter three- to five-pound set for triceps work, and a heavier five- to eight-pound set for everything else. We recommend two sets because, in general, the triceps muscles, or backs of the arms, will not be as strong as your biceps and shoulders when you're first starting out—so we target them using lighter weights until they gain strength and power. For any given exercise, your weights should be heavy enough that you are really feeling the burn by the end of the set. If you're not, your weights are too light and you need to go higher. We're not going to tell you it's okay to use soup cans or water bottles instead of weights because it's not—hopefully you are committed enough to this program and your health to invest in real weights to help you get the most out of the Warm-Up moves.

And now it's time to take a deep breath in and, as you exhale, leave the outside world and all your cares behind you. It's time to tune in to your body . . . this is your hour for you!

USING FREE WEIGHTS: A WORD ABOUT POSTURE

Maintaining good form or posture is essential for getting the most out of any exercise, but it's especially important when you're working with free weights. When you pick up your weights, be sure that you continue to stand tall with your shoulders back and your chest open; don't let your weights round your shoulders and pull you down. Even when you are directed to lean your torso forward, as with a move like Triceps Pressbacks, focus on keeping your spine straight and don't let those shoulders drop. Always think like a ballerina: Slouching isn't pretty!

KNEE LIFTS

A graceful alternative to the old-school march-in-place, this is one of the fastest ways to elevate your heart rate and prepare your body for the next 57 minutes. You're setting the pace and tone for your workout, so let's get those knees up!

MUSCLES TARGETED: *Entire body*

The Steps

- Stand tall and draw your navel toward your spine.

- Energetically push your right foot off the floor and lift your right knee up to hip level while swinging your left arm up and out in front of you.

- Now lower your left arm and right knee as you simultaneously raise the left knee and right arm. Continue to lift and lower knees and arms while alternating sides at a brisk tempo.

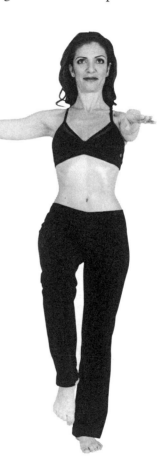

PHYSIQUE 57 TIP

With every lift, imagine that you are giving yourself a lift—reversing the effects of gravity and aging!

BICEPS CURLS

Biceps Curls continue your warm-up and jump-start your metabolic rate. Make sure you feel the burn—you'll love showing off those guns!

> MUSCLES TARGETED: *Biceps*
>
> WHAT YOU'LL NEED: *5- to 8-pound weights*

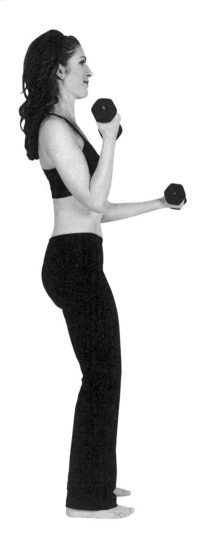

The Steps

- Pick up your weights and stand with your feet hip-width apart, knees slightly bent.

- Tuck your elbows into the sides of your body and rotate your arms so your palms are facing up. Draw your abdominal muscles in and drop your tailbone down. Imagine that your spine is lengthening behind you.

- Curl the right weight up toward your right shoulder and then lower it toward your thigh. As you lower the right weight, curl the left weight up to your left shoulder. Continue alternating at a smooth pace.

- Your elbows should stay at your sides the entire time.

HAMMER CURLS

Hammer Curls are just like Biceps Curls except that we rotate the position of the wrist to target the biceps from a different angle, ensuring that we hit and tone every single one of those muscle fibers. You'll be able to see your muscles working and gaining definition with every rep!

> MUSCLES TARGETED: *Biceps*
>
> WHAT YOU'LL NEED: *5- to 8-pound weights*

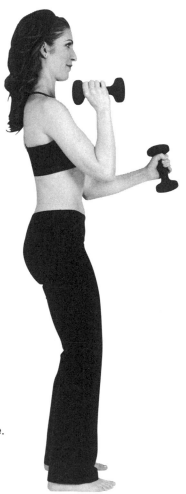

The Steps

- Pick up your weights and stand with your feet hip-width apart, knees slightly bent.

- Tuck your elbows into the sides of your body and rotate your arms so your palms are facing each other. Draw your abdominal muscles in and drop your tailbone down. Imagine that your spine is lengthening behind you.

- With your palms facing in, curl the right weight up toward your right shoulder and then lower it toward your thigh. As you lower the right weight, curl the left weight up to your left shoulder. Continue alternating at a smooth pace.

- Your elbows should stay at your sides the entire time.

PHYSIQUE 57 TIP
Don't be afraid of heavy weights—they are the secret to achieving a sexy, sculpted upper body!

SHOULDER PULSES

Shoulder Pulses keep your heart rate up and carve out the sexy, defined arms we all desire. This subtle move packs some serious sculpting punch—far better than the shoulder press machine at the gym!

> MUSCLES TARGETED: *Biceps, anterior deltoids*
>
> WHAT YOU'LL NEED: *5- to 8-pound weights*

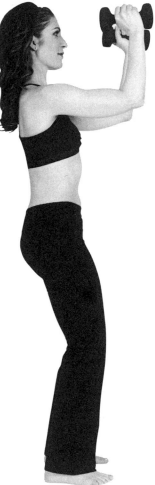

The Steps

- Pick up your weights and stand with your feet hip-width apart, knees slightly bent.

- With your palms facing in, bend your arms to a 90-degree angle and raise your elbows to slightly below shoulder level. Maintain the angle so that the weights remain directly above your elbows.

- Begin lifting your weights in small, upward pulses, making sure that your elbows never come above shoulder level.

- Draw your abdominal muscles in and keep your shoulders down. You want to feel as though your rib cage is drawn together in the front, like you're wearing a corset.

Note: If you have any rotator cuff issues, use lighter weights or no weights at all.

PHYSIQUE 57 TIP

Visualize what you want your muscles to look like—long and lean, no bulk!

ROWS

This move is a welcome alternative to the rowing-to-nowhere machine at the gym. With strong back muscles, you will stand taller and have better posture all day long without even thinking about it. Plus, who wants back fat?

> MUSCLES TARGETED: *Upper back, posterior deltoids*
>
> WHAT YOU'LL NEED: *5- to 8-pound weights*

The Steps

- Pick up your weights and step your feet wider than your hips, keeping your feet parallel.

- Bend your knees and lean forward from your hips at about a 45-degree angle. Keep your spine long from the crown of your head through your tailbone.

- With your palms facing each other, reach your arms forward and then, squeezing your shoulder blades together, bend your right elbow and bring the right weight all the way up next to your rib cage.

- As you extend the right weight back to the starting position, bring the left weight up to your rib cage. Continue alternating at a good pace.

- You want to keep your elbows close to your body as you row—feel them skimming along your waistline.

- Keep your abdominal muscles engaged the entire time to feel more of a burn!

> TO MODIFY: *Use lighter weights if necessary.*

ROWS WITH WIDE ELBOWS

This variation on traditional Rows targets your upper back and shoulder muscles from a different angle. If you like to wear strapless dresses, this is the move for you—your back muscles will look amazing. Nothing soft or hanging out!

> MUSCLES TARGETED: *Upper back, posterior deltoids*
>
> WHAT YOU'LL NEED: *5- to 8-pound weights*

The Steps

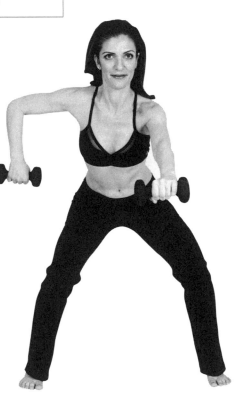

- Pick up your weights and step your feet wider than your hips, keeping your feet parallel.

- Bend your knees and lean forward from your hips at about a 45-degree angle. Keep your spine long from the crown of your head through your tailbone.

- With your palms facing down, thumbs toward each other, reach your arms forward and then, squeezing your shoulder blades together, bend your right elbow and bring it up in line with your right shoulder.

- As you extend the right weight back to starting position, bend your left elbow and bring it up in line with your left shoulder.

- Continue alternating at a smooth pace.

> TO MODIFY: *Use lighter weights if necessary.*

PHYSIQUE 57 TIP

Engage those abs! The way you work out is the way you design your body—if you hold your abs in for an hour, they will stay that way when you finish.

SCARECROWS

Scarecrows are a fabulous way to work both the triceps and the muscles in your upper back that you don't want hanging over your bra straps—what a combination!

MUSCLES TARGETED: *Triceps, upper back*

WHAT YOU'LL NEED: *3- to 5-pound weights*

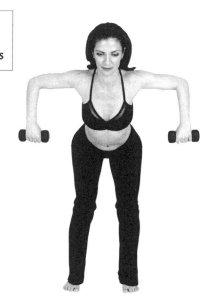

The Steps

- Pick up your lighter set of weights and stand with your feet hip-width apart, knees slightly bent.

- Draw your abdominal muscles in and lean your body forward at a 45-degree angle.

- Bend your elbows and bring them up and out to your sides in line with your shoulders—imagine a straight line drawn from one elbow across to the other. Your palms are facing behind you.

- Press the weights out until your arms are straight, and then bend them in again toward your chest.

- Relax your shoulders and keep your elbows lifted.

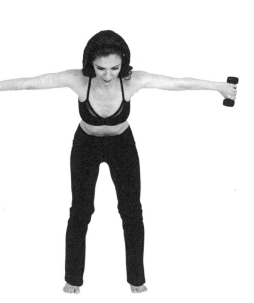

TO MODIFY: *Use lighter weights if necessary.*

TRICEPS PRESSBACKS

Our back-of-the-arm muscles are frequently flabby since they don't get much use in
everyday activities. But if you want to look sensational in tanks and sleeveless dresses,
firm triceps are a must. So grab your weights and use this exercise to press out the flab!

> MUSCLES TARGETED: *Triceps*
>
> WHAT YOU'LL NEED: *3- to 5-pound weights*

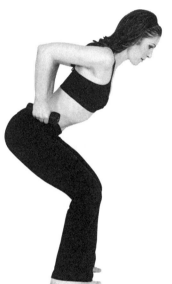

The Steps

- Pick up your lighter set of weights and stand with
  your feet hip-width apart, knees slightly bent.

- Draw your abdominal muscles in and lean your
  body forward at a 45-degree angle.

- Bring your weights to your hips so that your elbows
  are pointing behind you.

- Now press both of the weights out behind you,
  reaching your arms long and straight.

- Bend your elbows and bring your weights
  back to your hips.

- Be sure to relax your shoulders. Put the brakes on as
  you bring the weights back to your hips so you work
  the triceps on both the way up and the way down.

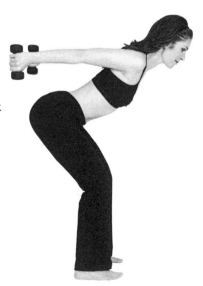

> TO MODIFY: *Use lighter weights
> if necessary.*

PHYSIQUE 57 TIP

Press away all those flabby areas—
muscle eats fat! Press, press, press!

PUSH-UPS

Push-Ups are empowering! In this classic but super-effective move, cardio and strength training come together as you start to stoke your metabolic rate. This full-body effort trims and tones you from head to toe with a special emphasis on shoulders, pecs, and abs. Plus, the lower you go, the less armpit fat you'll have.

MUSCLES TARGETED: *Entire body*

The Steps

- From a kneeling position, lean forward and place your hands on the floor a little wider than shoulder-width apart, fingers facing forward.

- Step your feet back and straighten your legs so that your body forms a straight line from your head to your feet. Keep your abdominal muscles engaged and your seat tight—don't let your belly droop toward the floor.

- Bend your elbows to lower your chest as far as you can toward the floor, and then push back up to straighten your arms.

- Use your abdominal muscles to keep your body long like a plank throughout this exercise.

TO MODIFY: *If you can't do a full-form Push-Up yet, you can modify by bending your knees, shifting your body weight forward onto your thighs, and bringing your heels close to your bottom. Build up your strength here and then give the full-form Push-Ups a shot!*

ADVANCED: *Try doing half the set with your right leg crossed on top of the left, and then switch. This increases the challenge for your core and your arms.*

PHYSIQUE 57 TIP

Remember, you can't think yourself into shape—if you want a great body, you have to work for it.

PLANK WITH LEG LIFTS

Connecting with your core while lifting your legs sculpts both the front and the back of your body—how efficient!

MUSCLES TARGETED: *Entire body*

The Steps

- Begin in a full-form Push-Up position (page 47) with your legs slightly apart.

- Soften your elbows slightly and strongly pull in your abdominal muscles to keep your hips in line with the rest of your body.

- Now lift your right leg off the floor and, keeping it straight and your toes pointed, pulse it upward toward the ceiling. This is a small, controlled movement—only about 2 or 3 inches. Continue pulsing at a good pace.

- Now switch sides.

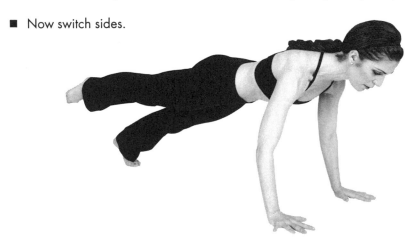

TO MODIFY: *Come down on your hands and knees. Keep the left knee on the floor as you extend and pulse your right leg, and then switch.*

PHYSIQUE 57 TIP

Don't be discouraged if you can't finish a set. You did five lifts, that's good—next time you'll do ten.

FOREARM PLANK

This is one of the best moves ever for toning your middle and revving up your metabolism. Resting on your forearms pushes you to engage your back and core muscles on a much deeper level and allows you to perform more multitasking variations than you can in a regular plank position. It requires a bit of concentration, but now is the time to really start bringing your body and mind together. Keep that abdominal wall tight!

MUSCLES TARGETED: *Entire body*

The Setup

- From a kneeling position, lean forward and place your forearms on the floor shoulder-width apart, with your palms facing down and your elbows directly underneath the shoulders. Keep your hips and torso off the floor.

- Press your legs back and straighten them as long as possible behind you while resting on your forearms for balance. Keep your abdominal wall tight and don't let your hips sink down. Your feet are flexed, toes pressing into the floor, and your neck is straight, in line with your spine. This is your starting position.

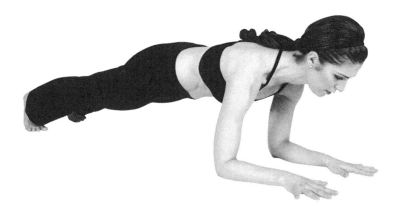

VARIATIONS

A. Alternating Knee Bends

- Keeping your toes on the floor, press through the balls of your feet and bend the right knee toward the floor, then the left—make sure they don't quite touch. Continue alternating knees while keeping your core stable.

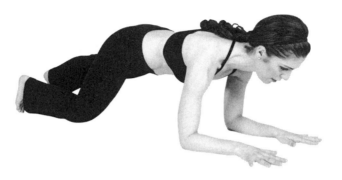

B. Both Knees Bending

- Keeping your toes on the floor, bend both knees down toward the floor—make sure they don't quite touch—and then extend back through your heels to straighten.

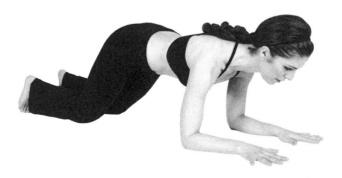

C. Both Knees Bending with Ball

- Place the playground ball between your inner thighs, squeezing it just enough to make it form an egg shape.

- Keeping your toes on the floor, bend your knees down toward the floor—make sure they don't quite touch—and then extend back through your heels to straighten while maintaining the squeeze on the ball. This variation provides a fabulous isometric challenge for your adductors—no more inner thigh flab!

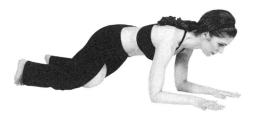

D. Hip Twists

- Twist your hips toward the floor, first to the right side, then the left. Imagine that you are drawing an arc with your hips: The movement you want is "up and over," not "side-to-side." Keep your forearms anchored on the floor.

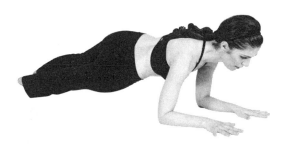

TO MODIFY: *If any of the variations are too challenging, you can hold the Forearm Plank position without any additional leg or hip movements.*

PHYSIQUE *57* TIP

Don't forget that your goal is to create a balanced body: one that is equal in strength and flexibility.

TRICEPS DIPS

We love any opportunity to target the backs of the arms! This move appears in the Warm-Up but is also sprinkled throughout your entire workout.

MUSCLES TARGETED: *Triceps*

The Steps

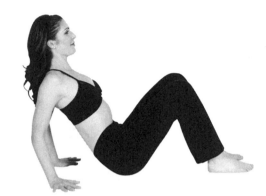

- Sit on the floor with your knees bent and your feet flat on the floor in front of you, about hip-width apart. Place your hands about 5 or 6 inches behind you with your fingertips facing forward.

- Lift your hips off the floor a few inches and shift your body weight back toward your hands.

- Now bend and straighten your elbows, concentrating the movement in your triceps. As you lift and lower, keep your elbows pointing back and do not lock your arms or let your seat touch the floor. Feel those triceps muscles quiver—wherever you feel the heat, you are making muscle!

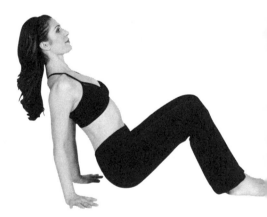

ADVANCED: *Straighten your legs and push your hips up.*

Note: If you have weak wrists, press into your knuckles with your thumbs facing toward your seat.

TRICEPS CAN-CAN

Working your triceps has never been so fun! In this move, cardio, isometrics, and strength training come together to launch you into your calorie-burning zone. You'll also be gaining flexibility in your hamstrings and strengthening your thighs and core. All of these benefits, plus super-toned triceps, make this move a winner.

> MUSCLES TARGETED: *Triceps, quadriceps, core*

The Steps

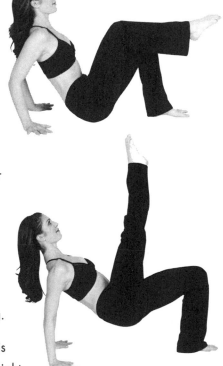

- Sit on the floor with your knees bent and your feet flat on the floor in front of you, about hip-width apart. Place your hands 5 to 6 inches behind you with your fingertips facing forward.

- Lift your hips off the floor a few inches and shift your body weight back toward your hands.

- Bend your right knee and bring it in toward your chest, bending your elbows as in Triceps Dips (page 52).

- Now straighten your arms, and simultaneously straighten your right leg toward the ceiling. Then bend your elbows and bend your right knee again. Keep on bending and straightening.

- Remember, when your elbows are bent, the leg is bent; when your arms are straight, the leg is straight.

- Try to find a heat-producing tempo. Now you look like a showgirl!

PHYSIQUE 57 TIP

Get inspired, get enthusiastic—you'll see better results!

TRICEPS STRETCH

This simple stretch lengthens your triceps after all those dips and pressbacks to create long, lean muscle. You'll look like a ballerina, not a bodybuilder!

> MUSCLES TARGETED: *Triceps*

The Steps

- Sit cross-legged on the floor with your abs pulled in and your spine tall.

- Raise your right arm up alongside your head and bend your elbow. Use your left hand to take hold of your right elbow.

- Pull the right elbow down and back behind your head to stretch your right triceps.

- Repeat this stretch on the left side.

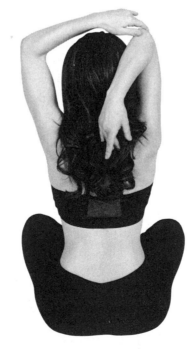

SHOULDER OPENER STRETCH

This stretch gives you energy and helps you to breathe better by expanding your entire chest and shoulder area. In addition to prepping you for your Thigh series, it helps you avoid a hunched posture—do it anytime your back and shoulders need perking up.

> MUSCLES TARGETED: *Pecs, shoulders*

The Steps

- Sit cross-legged on the floor with your abs pulled in and your spine tall.

- Bring both arms behind your body and clasp your hands together, palms touching.

- Now straighten your arms and extend them out and up, pressing your shoulders back as far as you can. You can lean forward slightly as you stretch.

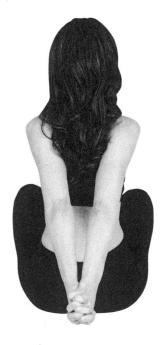

CHAPTER 4

THIGHS

NOW THAT YOUR METABOLIC RATE IS STOKED, WE WANT to keep you in the calorie-burning zone and take things up a notch. The next section of your workout is Thighs: the series where we blast away those saddlebags, knee flaps, and jiggly inner thighs and replace them with slim, toned, sexy legs that will make wearing shorts and miniskirts a pleasure. Our Thigh series is designed to get your heart muscle pumping and your thighs shaking, and that's just the way we like it—anything less than that is not worth it!

Your thighs are made up of four different major muscle groups: the quadriceps (the anterior, or front, of the thigh muscles), the hamstrings (the posterior, or back, of the thigh muscles), the adductors (inner thighs), and the abductors (outer thighs). Together they make up the single largest muscle group in the body, and they generate by far the biggest caloric burn—in fact, your quadriceps alone burn more calories than any other set of muscles. Thus we spend a lot of our time on thighs because we feel that this is where you can really make your gains: With every new series of reps, you are breaking down fat to fuel the thighs' major caloric burn, and sculpting the muscles themselves into powerhouses of lean tissue that will burn extra calories for you around the clock. Whereas most workouts tend to emphasize the quads and hamstrings—and the repetitive anterior-posterior movements that are the hallmarks of running, spinning, and aerobics—our moves are specifically designed to target ALL FOUR of the thighs' major muscle groups. Throughout our Thigh series, we're constantly tightening and tapering every single one of those hard-to-reach muscles: firming them up, pulling them in, and wrapping them ever closer to the bone.

The series is broken down into three separate sections. The first two are performed standing up and use a rapid-fire sequence of positions and variations to isolate and target the different muscles. At just four minutes apiece, these sections are perfectly timed to work your muscles to their max and then give you a chance to recover; if you continued working much longer than four minutes, your form would get sloppy and you'd see diminishing returns. So we perform the two sections back-to-back with a two-minute series of stretches in between: We hit all four areas hard—quads, hamstrings, abductors, adductors—then stretch and change positions and hit them all hard again in a different way. These sections complement one another and incorporate a wide variety of angles and ranges of movement, all the better to engage those tiny ancillary muscles, as well as the muscles in the lower leg, especially calves. We also use a playground ball in many of the moves to spot-target the inner thighs whenever we can and make sure they don't get overlooked. All in all, our thigh workout is kind of like a rotisserie: We're getting every muscle all around!

The third section is Thigh Dancing, which provides a fun way to sculpt your waistline and hips along with your thighs. For Thigh Dancing, we get down on the floor and really move and groove to the music, which can feel like a welcome break after all that standing thigh work. But make no mistake—Thigh Dancing is hard! We engage the entire thigh in an isometric hold and then perform pulses, tucks, and other micromovements designed to overload your muscles one more time and finish the job. Thigh Dancing is like having one last cocktail—after that, you're done and it's time to move on!

When it comes to the stretches, we do two different sets for thighs, each of which serves a slightly different purpose. The first set is performed right after the first Thigh section and is all about the recovery interval—we want to keep you in the fat-burning zone, so we move right through a brief series of stretches, giving your muscles a quick chance to recharge so that you can start the second

THIGH BOOSTERS:

Our Two Favorite Moves for Thighs

You can use these moves to supplement your workouts, or to sculpt your thighs whenever you have a few extra minutes:

- Thigh Dancing: 1½ minutes (page 80)
- Kick Line: 1 minute (page 78)

Thigh section even stronger. The second stretch series occurs after Thigh Dancing and provides a bit of a deeper stretch—we take more time, breathe more deeply, and really lengthen and soothe those muscles as we round out the thigh portion of the workout.

Our Thigh series is definitely the most cardio-intensive part of our workout, and many of the moves include arm movements and other elements designed to get your heart rate up and provide a burst of aerobic intensity. Therefore it's not surprising that many of our clients find this series to be their biggest challenge. But with great challenges come great rewards—and if you can do four minutes of Skier and Swivel Chair, or do one more set of Hip Tucks when your quads have turned to jelly, you'll know you can conquer anything in the outside world!

So now it's time to start feeling some heat and find your inner Thigh Warrior. When you feel those muscles start to shake and quiver, just keep thinking: MIND OVER THIGHS!

BEFORE YOU BEGIN...

The majority of the moves in this chapter require a waist-high chair or sturdy piece of furniture for support. Before you begin, please check to be sure that your furniture is stable. If necessary, place the heavy set of weights from your warm-up on your chair for additional stability.

SMALL V

A hip take on classical ballet's first position, our Small V series offers a whole new way of trimming your thighs. Variations such as pulses and hip shakes get you right into your calorie-burning zone and start slimming away those extra inches.

MUSCLES TARGETED: *Quadriceps*

WHAT YOU'LL NEED: *A waist-high, sturdy piece of furniture; a playground ball*

The Setup

- Stand facing your furniture about a fore-arm's distance away and hold on to it with your hands apart, slightly wider than your shoulders.

- Make a small V with your feet by bringing your heels together. Your big toes should be 2 or 3 inches apart.

- Keeping your heels together, raise them up a couple of inches off the floor. Keep your spine straight and feel all ten toes pressing evenly into the floor.

- Now bend your knees and lower your body to a challenging level—the place where you feel your thigh muscles engaged—about 5 or 6 inches down. This is your starting position.

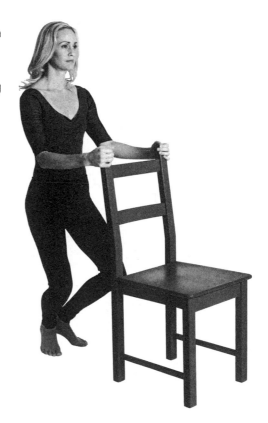

VARIATIONS

A. Pulses

■ Bend your knees deeper and begin to perform small pulses, up and down. Remember, this is a small, controlled movement—only about 2 or 3 inches. Look straight ahead and keep your abdominal muscles pulled in so that your tailbone is pointing toward your heels. You should feel a lot of heat throughout your thighs and be able to easily maintain your balance. Remember: Don't come up past your starting position.

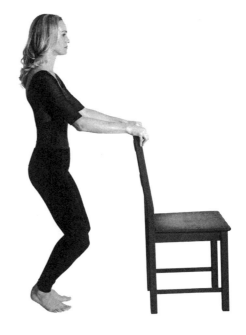

B. Hip Tucks

■ Keeping your upper body straight, roll your hips forward and then release them back. Again, these Hip Tucks are small, controlled movements: Your legs remain steady, your heels off the floor. And keep those knees bent—you didn't come up, did you?

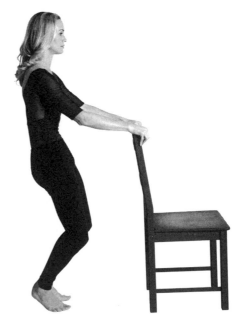

C. Seat to Heels and Up

- This is a larger range of movement. Bend your knees and glide straight down until your tailbone hovers above your heels, and then come right back up to your starting position. Remember to keep your heels together the entire time, and make sure your knees are tracking over your toes and not opening out to the sides. When you lower, you want to feel like your spine is gliding along a wall behind you, so that your heels, hips, and shoulders are all aligned. Here you should be building a lot of heat and really feeling your heart muscle working!

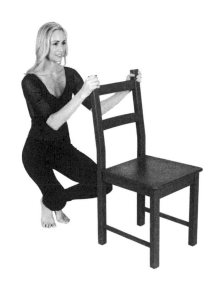

D. Seat to Heels and Up with Ball

- Place the playground ball between your inner thighs, squeezing it just enough to form an egg shape.

- Bend your knees and glide straight down until your tailbone hovers above your heels, then come right back up to your starting position. Remember to keep your heels together the entire time and maintain the squeeze on the ball.

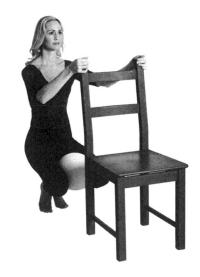

E. Hip Shakes

■ Shake your hips first right, then left. Again, this is a small, controlled movement rather than a loose shake—your upper body remains still. Rather than swinging your hips wildly from side to side, you want to lift them up toward your shoulders by using your obliques—the muscles that lie along the sides of your torso and help to define your waistline. Pretend there's a kickstand underneath your heels so they remain in position, not moving.

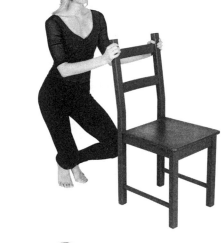

F. Hip Circles

■ Roll your hips forward, right, back, and left to make a complete circle. Keep your knees and shoulders as still as possible and concentrate the movement in your hips. Imagine that you are carving the circle carefully, deliberately, always maintaining control. This variation gets a lot of heat going in your abs!

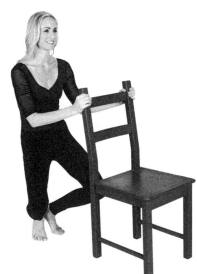

ADVANCED: *You can always stay lower in this position!*

Note: If you have any knee issues, stay up higher in the position.

PHYSIQUE 57 TIP

Whenever you feel the heat, you are making muscle. If you're not feeling it, what you're doing isn't working.

SMALL V INCLINE

This variation on Small V changes the angle of the spine to enable you to go farther and work deeper into your thigh muscles. We keep the calorie burn on high and make sure you're achieving overload at every possible angle. This position also engages more of the core—an added bonus.

MUSCLES TARGETED: *Quadriceps, hamstrings, calves, core*

WHAT YOU'LL NEED: *A waist-high, sturdy piece of furniture*

The Setup

- Stand facing your furniture, about a forearm's distance away, and hold on to it with your hands apart, slightly wider than your shoulders. Your feet are in Small V position: heels together, big toes 2 to 3 inches apart.

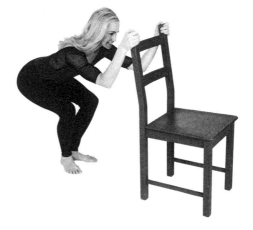

- Holding on to your piece of furniture, bend your knees and incline your chest forward so your spine is at a 45-degree angle, then lower your seat as close to knee level as possible. Your arms are bent and remain bent while lowering; your feet are flat on the floor; your knees are over your ankles; and your neck and spine remain straight. This is your starting position.

VARIATIONS

A. Pulses

- Bend your knees deeper and begin performing small pulses, up and down. Remember, this is a small, controlled movement—only about 2 or 3 inches. Your knees should remain anchored over your ankles throughout the movement. Maintain the angle of the torso and keep your feet flat.

B. Seat Toward Heels and Up

- Raise your heels up off the floor so that you're on the balls of your feet.

- Keeping your heels together, bend your knees deeply and lower your seat as far as you can toward your heels while maintaining the angle of your torso. Make sure your knees are tracking over your toes and not opening out to the sides. Then come back up to your starting position.

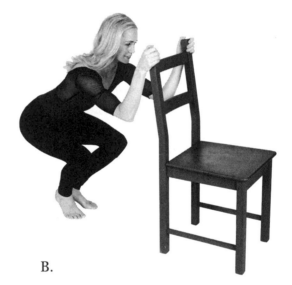

B.

PHYSIQUE 57 TIP

Your thighs are your calorie-burning muscles. Ask yourself: *How many calories do I want to burn today?*

POWER PLIÉ WITH BALL

The Power Plié series is a fabulous alternative to jump squats that will smooth your thigh muscles and create major definition. As a bonus, holding the playground ball isometrically tones your shoulders and arms while engaging the muscles in the core. In this position, you'll really feel the cardio aspect of your workout and be able to increase your endurance and stamina. Push deeper into the Power Plié to find your inner Thigh Warrior!

MUSCLES TARGETED: *Quadriceps, hamstrings, abductors, calves, obliques*

WHAT YOU'LL NEED: *A playground ball*

The Setup

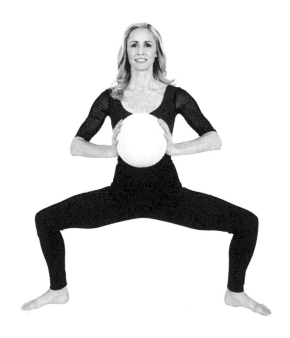

- Step away from your furniture and take a wide stance, holding the playground ball in your hands. Your feet should turn out naturally from your hips—don't force it—and be wide enough apart that you can lower your hips to knee level.

- Keeping your torso upright, bend your knees and bring your hips down to knee level.

- Now squeeze the ball between your palms at chest level, keeping your elbows wide to the side. This is your starting position.

VARIATIONS

A. Pulses

- Bend your knees deeper and begin to perform small pulses, up and down. Remember, this is a small, controlled movement—only about 2 or 3 inches. Your hips should stay right around knee level the entire time.

- Make sure you feel all four corners of each foot pressing evenly into the floor—you don't want to be rocking toward your insteps (if you are, turn your feet slightly in).

- As you pulse, think about getting deeper and lower in your legs, but taller through your torso—keep your posture working for you!

B. Hip Tucks

- Roll your hips forward and then release them back. Be sure that your knees remain anchored. Don't let them rock back and forth—keep the movement in your hips. You'll really feel this in your adductor muscles, especially if you press into your heels. Bye-bye, jiggly inner thighs!

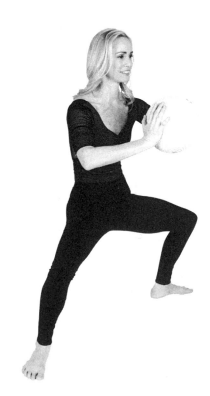

B.

C. Hip Shakes

- Shake your hips first right, then left. This should be a small, controlled movement rather than a loose shake—your upper body remains still, and you use your obliques to lift your hips up toward your shoulders.

- Be sure that your knees remain anchored. Don't let them rock back and forth—keep the movement in your hips. Make sure that all four corners of each foot are pressing evenly into the floor.

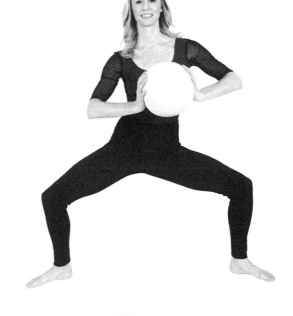

D. Hip Circles

- Roll your hips forward, right, back, and left to make a complete circle. Keep your knees and shoulders as still as possible and concentrate the movement in your hips. Imagine that you are carving the circle carefully, deliberately, always maintaining control.

- Be sure that your knees remain anchored. Don't let them rock back and forth—keep all four corners of each foot pressing evenly into the floor.

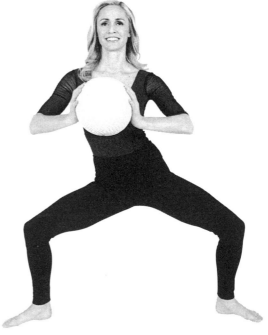

E. Alternate Heel Raises with Pulses

- Raise the ball up over your head and hold it there, keeping your arms and spine straight.

- Begin pulsing. Keeping the rhythmic tempo, begin lifting your heels off the floor, first right, then left, so that every time you are pulsing down, one heel is up and one heel is down.

- Keep your torso steady and don't drop the ball! This is where cardio and strength training come together—do you feel overloaded now?

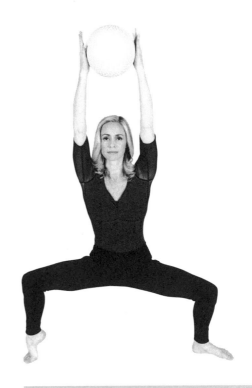

Note: To modify, or if you have knee issues, keep your hips higher than your knees.

PHYSIQUE 57 TIP

Endurance changes the shape of your body. What you put in, you will get back out!

SKIER

Like the Small V Incline, this position enables you to go farther and deeper into your thigh work by changing the angle of the spine. With your feet parallel and your legs together, you engage the entire backs of your legs as well as your core. No more endless, boring squats—instead, imagine that you are flying down the slopes of the Swiss Alps: light, graceful, and amazingly strong!

> MUSCLES TARGETED: *Quadriceps, hamstrings, calves, core*
>
> WHAT YOU'LL NEED: *A waist-high, sturdy piece of furniture*

The Setup

- Stand facing your furniture, about a forearm's distance away, and hold on to it with your hands apart, slightly wider than your shoulders. Squeeze your feet, knees, and thighs together, side by side.

- Holding on to your piece of furniture, bend your knees and incline your chest forward so your spine is at a 45-degree angle, then lower your seat as close to knee level as possible. Your arms are bent and remain bent while lowering; your feet are flat on the floor; your knees are over your ankles; your neck and spine remain straight. This is your starting position.

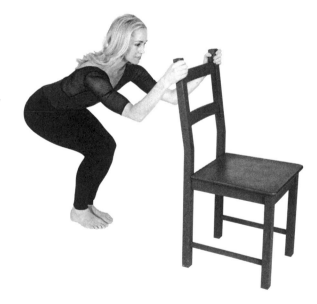

VARIATIONS

A. Pulses

- Bend your knees deeper and begin to perform small pulses, up and down. Remember, this is a small, controlled movement—only about 2 or 3 inches. Your knees should remain anchored over your ankles throughout the movement. Maintain the angle of the torso.

B. Seat Toward Heels and Up

- Raise your heels a couple of inches off the floor so that you are on the balls of your feet.

- Bend your knees deeply and lower your seat as far as you can toward your heels while maintaining the angle of your torso. Keep your inner thighs glued together as you lower and lift. Then come back up to your starting position.

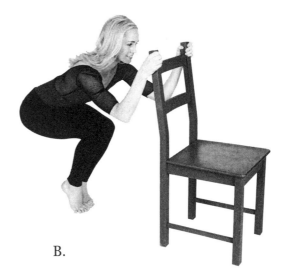

B.

PHYSIQUE 57 TIP

Watch your posture—when your body is in alignment, everything else will fall into place.

SKIER WITH BALL

This ultra-challenging version of Skier is one of the most unique ways to tone and sculpt all four areas of your thighs. By adding the playground ball, you'll be zeroing in on those hard-to-hit adductor muscles, or inner thighs. If you're tired of feeling your thighs brush together when you walk, this is the move for you— skinny jeans and leggings will be your friends!

MUSCLES TARGETED: *Quadriceps, hamstrings, adductors, calves, core*

WHAT YOU'LL NEED: *A waist-high, sturdy piece of furniture; a playground ball*

The Setup

- Stand facing your furniture, about a forearm's distance away, and hold on to it with your hands apart, slightly wider than your shoulders. Place your feet in a parallel position on the floor, about hip-width apart.

- Now place the ball between your thighs. Your feet should remain parallel. You want enough of a squeeze on the ball to make the ball into an egg shape.

- Holding on to your piece of furni-ture, bend your knees and incline your chest forward so your spine is at a 45-degree angle. Then lower your seat toward knee level. Your arms are bent and remain bent while lowering; your knees are over your ankles; your feet are flat; your neck and spine remain straight. This is your start-ing position.

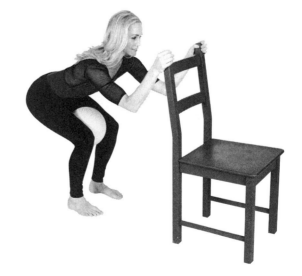

VARIATIONS

A. Squeezes on the Ball

- Squeeze your inner thighs into the ball and then release. This is a deliberate, controlled movement; keep your knees anchored over your ankles.

B. Seat Toward Heels and Up

- Raise your heels up inches off the floor so that you are on the balls of your feet.

- Bend your knees deeply and lower your seat as far as you can toward your heels while maintaining the angle of your torso. Then come back up to your starting position. Maintain the squeeze on the ball throughout.

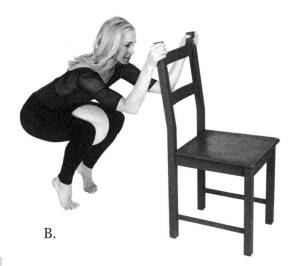

B.

PHYSIQUE 57 TIP

Always remember, you can design your own body. You are the sculptor; you are in charge.

SWIVEL CHAIR

We love this exercise for you! Swivel Chair keeps your core engaged while working your inner and outer thighs closer to the bone. Make sure you keep your thighs together throughout the move—that's a major challenge!

MUSCLES TARGETED: *Thighs, waistline*

WHAT YOU'LL NEED: *A waist-high, sturdy piece of furniture*

The Setup

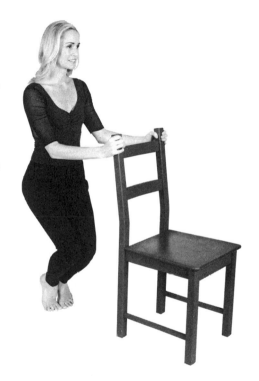

- Stand a forearm's distance away, facing your furniture with your feet, knees, and thighs together. Place your hands on your furniture a bit wider than shoulder-width apart.

- Keeping your upper body facing forward, rotate both feet and hips to point in the direction of your right hand (in the workouts, we'll do both sides).

- Lift your heels a couple of inches off the floor and bend your knees to a challenging level—about 5 or 6 inches down. Keep your shoulders squared forward and your feet and thighs together. This is your starting position.

VARIATIONS

A. Pulses

- Bend your knees deeper and begin to perform small pulses, up and down. Remember, this is a small, controlled movement—only about 2 or 3 inches. Look straight ahead and keep your abdominal muscles pulled in so that your body weight stays forward and your tailbone is pointing toward your heels.

B. Hip Tucks

- Keeping your upper body still, roll your hips forward and then release them back. Again, these Hip Tucks are small, controlled movements. Your legs remain in your starting position: knees and thighs together, tailbone over your heels, and heels off the floor.

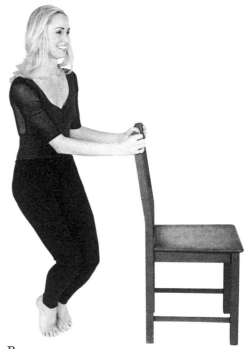

B.

C. Seat to Heels and Up

- Bend your knees deeply and lower your torso so that you hover a few inches above your heels. Then come back up to the starting position. Your upper body should face forward throughout the movement, and if your knees start to separate as you get closer to your heels, be sure to bring them back together on the way up. You'll really feel the burn with this one—but remember: MIND OVER THIGHS!

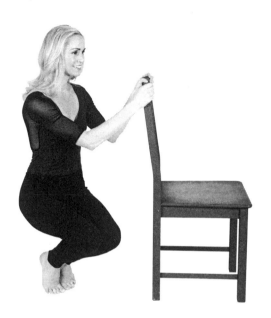

ADVANCED: *Bend your knees deeper in your starting position.*

Note: To modify, or if you have weak knees, you can always stay up higher in this position—we promise you'll still feel the burn!

PHYSIQUE 57 TIP

Pulsing is your friend—if you start to fall apart, at least keep pulsing so you stay in the calorie-burning zone.

CURTSY

A great alternative to the boring abductor machine at the gym, the Curtsy works your inner and outer thighs at the same time, slimming away saddlebags and thunder thighs for lean, shapely legs. It also builds core strength and makes you feel feminine and graceful. Besides, you never know when you'll need to curtsy!

> MUSCLES TARGETED: *Inner and outer thighs, core*
>
> WHAT YOU'LL NEED: *A waist-high, sturdy piece of furniture*

The Setup

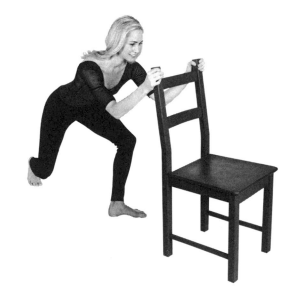

- Standing a forearm's distance away, face your furniture and hold on to it with your hands slightly wider than shoulder-width apart. Step your feet into a Small V position: heels together, big toes 2 to 3 inches apart.

- Holding on to your piece of furniture, incline your chest forward at a 45-degree angle.

- Bend your knees and cross your right foot behind you toward your left shoulder, placing the ball of your foot on the floor (in the workouts, we'll do both sides).

- Now bend both knees deeply. Your right knee should hover a few inches off the floor, so step your right foot farther back if necessary. Your feet and knees should be slightly turned out; keep the left foot flat. This is your starting position.

VARIATIONS

A. Pulses

- Bend your knees deeper and lower and lift your body in small, controlled movements, about 2 to 3 inches. Your chest remains inclined forward throughout the movement.

B. Single Leg Pulse

- Keeping your hips in place, lift the right leg off the floor and bring your right heel in toward your seat. This engages the seat and hamstring muscles.

- Now pulse the standing leg, bending your left knee to lower and lift your body in small, controlled movements, about 2 or 3 inches. Keep your abs tight to engage the core.

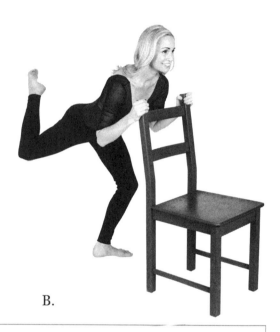

B.

ADVANCED: *Take your hands off the furniture and place them on your lower back.*

Note: If you have bad knees, do not go as low and do not turn your legs out as much.

PHYSIQUE 57 TIP

It's okay to quiver and shake—that's how you know you've found your edge.

KICK LINE

This is really a ballet move, and an amazingly healthy one at that: You are simultaneously lengthening and strengthening your muscles, while building bone density in your standing leg and strengthening your knee joints (a plus for anyone who has weak knees). Best of all, you can immediately feel your leg muscles becoming more defined. A welcome alternative to lunges, our Kick Line series will make you feel like a dancer—and give you the long, lithe legs to match!

> MUSCLES TARGETED: *Quadriceps*
>
> WHAT YOU'LL NEED: *A waist-high, sturdy piece of furniture*

The Setup

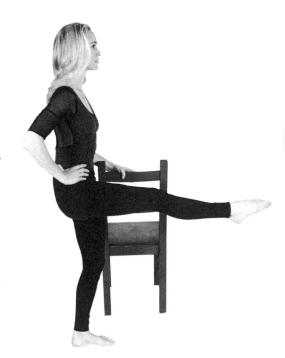

- Stand with your furniture on your left side and place your left hand on the furniture for balance (in the workouts, we'll do both sides).

- Lift and straighten your right leg out in front of you as high as you can (anywhere from 45 to 90 degrees off the floor is fine) while maintaining a tall, strong posture. Point your toes and keep your right knee facing the ceiling.

- Soften your standing leg by bending the knee slightly. This is your starting position.

- Remember, it's not about how high you can get the leg—you're not auditioning for the Rockettes, so don't sacrifice your form. Keep your abs tight and your spine long, reaching up through the crown of your head.

VARIATIONS

. . . .

A. Pulses

- Keeping your toes pointed, raise and lower your right leg about 2 to 3 inches in small, controlled movements. Keep your abs tight and your torso straight.

B. Grande Battement

- Tap your right toes down to the floor and then lift back up to your starting position. Make sure your toes remain pointed.

C. Microbend with Flexed Foot

- Flex the right foot and bend your right knee slightly, then press it back out to the starting position. Your torso remains straight.

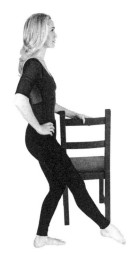

B.

> ADVANCED: *Raise the heel of your standing leg—this provides an additional workout for your standing calf muscle and extra protection against cankles!*

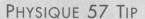

PHYSIQUE 57 TIP

Find your courage! Be a Thigh Warrior!

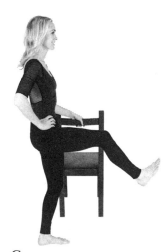

C.

THIGH DANCING

If you're at a party, pull this one out! One of our signature moves, Thigh Dancing is a fun, quick, and easy way to sculpt your thighs and stoke your metabolic rate. This unique exercise eliminates knee flaps—that sagging skin above the knee—and gives you more confidence when wearing shorts and skirts.

> MUSCLES TARGETED: *Quadriceps, core*
>
> WHAT YOU'LL NEED: *A mat or carpet under your knees*

The Setup

- Sit on your heels in a kneeling position. Your knees should be a few inches apart.

- Lift your seat a few inches off your heels. Keep your torso upright with your hands on your hips. This is your starting position.

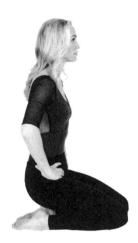

VARIATIONS

A. Hip Tucks

- Keeping your seat off your heels, roll your hips forward and then release them back. Push your arms out in front of you as you tuck.

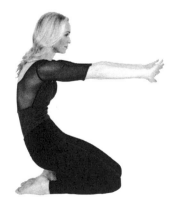

B. Hip Shakes

- Keeping your seat off your heels, shake your hips first right, then left. This is a small, controlled movement rather than a loose shake—you want to use your obliques to lift your hips up toward your shoulders rather than swinging them wildly from side to side.

- Bring your arms above your head and start to alternate pulling each elbow down—first one, then the other—as you shake your hips. By actively engaging your obliques, you are also whittling your waistline!

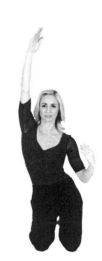

C. Hip Circles

- Keeping your seat off your heels, roll your hips forward, right, back, and left to make a complete circle. This movement is all in your hips: Imagine that you are carving the circle carefully, deliberately, always maintaining control.

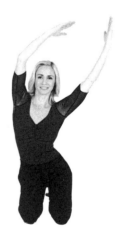

ADVANCED: *Keep your arms extended above your head the entire time.*

Note: If you have a knee injury, place an extra cushion under your knees and keep your seat higher above your heels. You can also use your arms in other fun ways during this move: Wave them side-to-side, do a lasso overhead—use your own creative license! Just make sure you maintain the core position throughout the movement.

PHYSIQUE 57 TIP

Firm up your core! If you don't feel it, pull it in harder!

THIGH DANCING WITH BALL

This sassy version of Thigh Dancing uses a playground ball to further engage the inner thighs, and girl-power arm movements to add a burst of cardio. Get on the calorie-burning freight train and go for it!

> MUSCLES TARGETED: *Quadriceps, adductors, core*
>
> WHAT YOU'LL NEED: *A mat or carpet under your knees; a playground ball*

The Setup

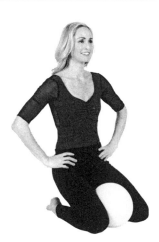

- Sit on your heels in a kneeling position. Place the playground ball between your inner thighs, squeezing it just enough to form an egg shape.

- Lift your seat a few inches off your heels. Keep your torso upright with your hands on your hips. This is your starting position.

VARIATIONS

A. Pulses Off Heels

- Using your thigh muscles, lift and lower your torso in small, controlled movements, about 2 or 3 inches. When you lower, come back to your starting position—don't sit back down on your heels.

B. Hand Jive

- Extend your arms straight out in front of you at chest level. Make fists with both hands.

■ Now rapidly crisscross your arms over
each other, first right over left, then
left over right. Keep going as quickly
as you can while maintaining control,
and don't sink back on your heels! Arm
crosses build heat and add a burst of
cardio to this move, while your thighs
remain engaged, clinging ever closer
to the bone.

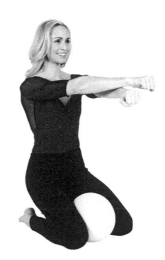

C. Boxer Girl

■ Make fists with both hands and bend
your arms in close to your body, keeping your elbows tucked into your sides.

■ Now perform Hip Shakes side-to-side while
punching your arms out at shoulder level,
alternating right and left. This works your
arm muscles as well as your thighs and
waistline. How fierce are you??

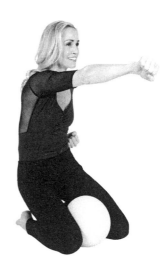

PHYSIQUE *57* TIP
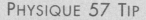
Make the attempt—as long as you
attempt, your body WILL change!

STANDING QUAD STRETCH

This stretch lengthens and relaxes your quads, giving them a brief period of recovery so that you can start your second Thigh section even stronger.

MUSCLES TARGETED: *Quadriceps*

WHAT YOU'LL NEED: *A waist-high, sturdy piece of furniture*

The Steps

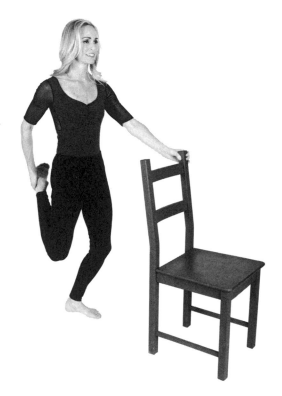

- Stand facing your furniture. Hold on to it with your left hand for balance.

- Bend your right knee to bring your right foot up behind you. With your right hand, take hold of the foot and pull it in toward your right seat muscle. Bend your standing leg slightly, and let the right knee point toward the floor as you feel a nice, long stretch through your quad.

- Try not to let your right leg flare out to the side—you want to keep it parallel to your standing leg to get the maximum benefit from this stretch.

- Repeat on the other side.

HAMSTRING STRETCH

A familiar ballet barre move, this stretch lengthens and relaxes your hamstrings before you start your second Thigh section.

> MUSCLES TARGETED: *Hamstrings, calves*
>
> WHAT YOU'LL NEED: *A waist-high, sturdy piece of furniture*

The Steps

■ Stand facing your furniture and take a large step back. Then lift your right leg and let the heel rest on top of the furniture.

■ Make sure that your standing foot is directly below your hips and that your hips are level (one isn't higher than the other).

■ Flex your right heel to get a deeper stretch all the way through your hamstring and your calf—you want to extend the back of your leg as long as you can.

■ If you want to go deeper into the stretch, fold your body forward over your right leg, reaching your tailbone behind you. Breathe deeply here!

■ Repeat on the other side.

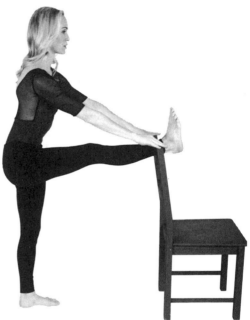

KNEELING STRETCH

This is a great, soothing release for your quads after Thigh Dancing, as well as a good hip and shoulder opener. You just want to lean back and gaze at your slimmer, sexier thighs. Can you see the heat coming off those muscles?

MUSCLES TARGETED: *Quadriceps, hip flexors*

WHAT YOU'LL NEED: *A mat or carpet under your knees*

The Steps

- Kneel on the floor with your knees hip-width apart and your legs slightly separated. Your seat should be resting on your heels.

- Place your palms on the floor behind you with your fingertips facing forward.

- Lift your seat up off your heels as far as you can go to feel the stretch along your quadriceps. Relax your neck and shoulders back and lift your chest toward the ceiling. Breathe deeply.

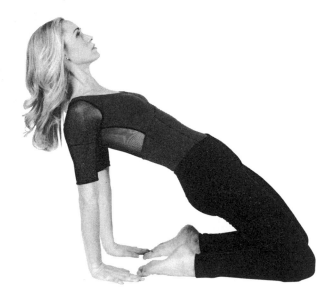

GAZELLE STRETCH

This elegant pose follows your Kneeling Stretch and provides a wonderful, lengthening release for your quads, hamstrings, and hip flexors. Lengthening the hip flexors also keeps your hips mobile and supple, which is essential for maintaining a youthful body.

MUSCLES TARGETED: *Quadriceps, hamstrings, hip flexors*

The Steps

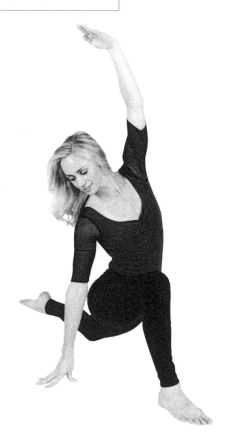

- From a kneeling position, step your right foot forward into a deep lunge, placing your right hand beside you on the floor for support. Shift your weight all the way forward to bring your right knee directly over your right ankle so you feel a nice, deep stretch through your hips—do not allow the knee to veer left or right. Relax your back foot.

- Now reach the left arm up over your head, and reach to the right to stretch your left side all the way down to your lower back.

- Repeat on the other side.

ANATOMICALLY CORRECT SPLIT

We like this split better than the typical Cheerleader Split because it gives you more bang for your buck: With our split, you keep your hips squared, which allows you to stretch your hip flexors as well as the hamstrings—a great multitasking move that is far better for your body.

MUSCLES TARGETED: *Hamstrings, hip flexors*

The Steps

- Coming out of your Gazelle Stretch, place both hands on the floor in front of you.

- Straighten your right knee and move your hips back toward the left foot. Don't sit down all the way, however—your seat should remain off the ground. Press your hands into the floor for stability.

- Keep your hips square and lower as far as you can—to your point of resistance. Point through your feet. Breathe deeply.

- Repeat on the other side.

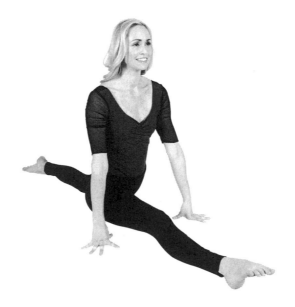

5

SEAT

GLUTEUS MAXIMUS, MEDIUS, MINIMUS…THESE ARE A FEW of our favorite things, and the Seat series targets them all. For many women, the seat and hips are the most challenging parts of the body to transform because, thanks to genetics, they tend to be where we store the most fat. Every fitness regimen targets the gluteus maximus—the two large muscles that form the curve of your buttocks—but we believe that you need to work far more than just your glutes if you want to achieve a shapely, lifted seat. So our Seat series is specifically designed to blast away fat by turning up the heat to boost your caloric burn, while going deep into *all* the major gluteal muscles, along with the dozens of tiny muscles in the hip and seat areas that will give you a firm, sexy, bikini-ready bottom.

The first half of our Seat series is performed standing up while holding on to a chair or sturdy piece of furniture. For each move, we start by engaging the seat, thigh, and core muscles in an isometric hold. Engaging the core is especially important during standing seat work, because it allows you to keep your hips still and create resistance for the gluteal muscles. If you don't brace your abs, you will lose the contraction in your glutes as soon as you start to move your legs. You might feel the muscles a little bit, but you won't be able to activate them to the degree that you would if your abs were pulled in tight. So the main thing you need to remember with standing seat work is to ALWAYS engage your abdominal muscles!

From there, we go on to perform sets of high-intensity variations that chisel and sculpt the seat through *abduction* movements. These are movements that engage the hip and seat muscles by lifting the leg out and away from the body at different angles. Our abduction movements are incredibly effective because they target the three major gluteal muscles all at once and force you to activate additional muscles throughout the body to stabilize the standing leg and control the range of movement. Our Speed Skater variation ups the ante by combining abduction with *adduction*, which means bringing the working leg in across the midline of the body. Speed Skater is a fabulous multitasking move that generates the most heat of any of the variations—you're digging deep into both the right AND the left glutes while activating the inner and outer hip muscles, core, and thighs, and mobilizing fat cells for some serious caloric burn. With all of these exercises, you'll also really feel the heat in your standing leg. And because standing, or weight-bearing, exercises improve bone density, your bones will be gaining strength as well—another plus!

For the second half of the series, we get down on the floor and target the same muscles again from a different angle. After pushing so hard with the standing work, moving to the floor can feel like a relief—but you'll find that simply changing positions gives you a whole new burst of energy that will enable you to keep going. In floor work, you don't have to engage the core quite as much, and the positioning is more straightforward. But changing the angle of the spine actually allows you to go deeper into the muscles—when you're not thinking about your posture or standing leg, you can really drill into all those seat muscles, large and small, with a laser-like precision and focus. By the time you reach the second seat stretch, you will have taken every single one of those muscles to the point of overload—and you will be on your way to a perfect, perky derriere with that coveted dimple on the side.

Our Seat series is intended to be ultra-challenging, so don't be discouraged if you can't make it through a full set of reps for some of the variations the first few times you try. You might have to pause in the middle of the set to do a quick stretch or shake out your legs and glutes before jumping back in. That's okay! You will feel a lot of burn and a lot of heat, but remember: That feeling is MUSCLE CHANGING! Cellulite doesn't like these moves, and all those tiny seat muscles will respond.

So take a deep breath and get ready to start slimming and sculpting that seat. If you need a little inspiration, let desire drive you through this portion of the workout: What do you desire? A lifted bottom!

SEAT BOOSTERS:

Our Two Favorite Moves for the Seat

You can use these moves to supplement your workouts, or to firm up your seat muscles whenever you have a few extra minutes:

- Pretzel: 1 minute (page 102)
- Hairpin: 1 minute (page 106)

STANDING CRANE

Say good-bye to the butt-blaster machine—this move is designed to sculpt your bottom and eliminate flab where your bottom meets your thighs. You always want to keep the working leg behind you in this exercise—find that perfect angle and muscle contraction once, and then keep firing away from there!

> MUSCLES TARGETED: *Gluteus maximus, medius, and minimus; hamstrings*
>
> WHAT YOU'LL NEED: *A waist-high, sturdy piece of furniture*

The Setup

- Facing your furniture, stand about a forearm's distance away and hold on to it with hands a bit wider than shoulder-width apart. Your elbows should be slightly bent.

- Lean your chest forward toward your hands, and bend both knees slightly.

- Bring your right heel up toward your right seat muscle and point your toes (in the workouts, we'll do both sides).

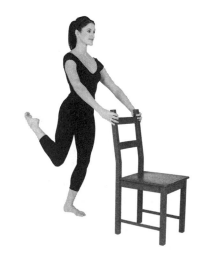

■ Now bring your right leg back so that your knee is facing toward the floor. Tip your tailbone slightly forward and engage your abs. This is your starting position.

VARIATIONS

A. Pulses to the Side

■ Keeping your toes pointed, raise your right leg 2 to 3 inches out to the side and then lower it again in small, controlled movements. Your hips should remain still and facing forward so the movement is isolated in your right gluteal muscles—don't let your hips rock or swing from side to side.

B. Press Leg Back

■ Keeping your knee bent, raise your right leg 2 to 3 inches out to the side, and flex your foot.

■ Keeping the heel close to your seat, press the right leg back about 2 or 3 inches in small, controlled movements. Again, this movement should be isolated in your seat muscles— your hips should not move. Keep your abdominal muscles drawn in and your spine long.

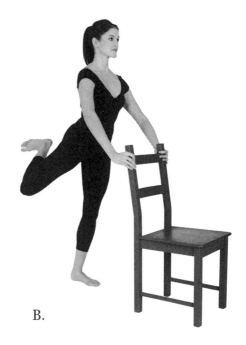

B.

C. Speed Skater

- Keeping your hips squared, point your toes and lift your right leg out to the side as high as you can while maintaining your form.

- Now cross your right knee behind your left knee as you bend the left knee deeper. Keep the right heel close to your seat as you lower. Then straighten your left leg and lift your right leg back up and return it to its highest point.

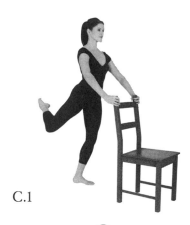

C.1

- This is a terrific move that generates the most heat out of all the variations—you're digging deep into the right AND left glutes for supercharged results.

D. Leg Circles

- Keeping your toes pointed and your heel close to your seat, draw a circle the size of a tennis ball with your right knee. Look at you, you're circling away cellulite!

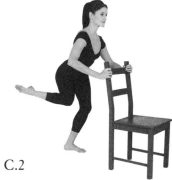

C.2

ADVANCED: *Place and squeeze the ball behind your bent knee throughout the exercise.*

PHYSIQUE 57 TIP

If you want to be chiseled, you've got to feel the heat. The more heat in your muscles, the more those fat cells can't stand it!

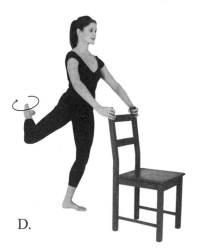

D.

FIGURE SKATER

It's time to push those seat muscles into overload! Feel the burn and keep your focus on a firmer flank—this series of moves will help you carve out that coveted indentation on the side of your seat.

MUSCLES TARGETED: *Entire seat, hamstrings, obliques*

WHAT YOU'LL NEED: *A waist-high, sturdy piece of furniture*

The Setup

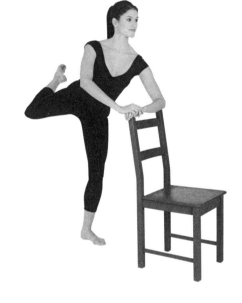

- Stand with your furniture on your left side (in the workouts, we'll do both sides). Lean sideways to place your left forearm on the furniture, keeping your hips in line with your elbow. Now take a big step away from the furniture so that your torso lengthens on an incline. You can place your right hand on the furniture in front of your left hand for additional support.

- Make sure your left foot is directly below your hips (pointing slightly toward your furniture) and soften that knee.

- Raise your right leg up to hip level and straighten it directly out to your side so that your body forms a T shape. Now bend your right knee about 90 degrees so that your heel moves toward your seat. Keep the right foot a little higher than your knee and keep your toes pointed. Remember to engage your abs. This is your starting position.

VARIATIONS

· · · · · · · · · · · · · · · · · · · ·

A. Pulses to the Side

- Lift and lower your right leg about 2 or 3 inches in small, controlled movements using the muscles in the side of your seat—you'll feel these kick in right away! Try not to let the leg swing forward; keep your toes pointed and your right thigh in line with your torso.

B. Press Leg Back

- Now flex your foot and press the right leg back behind you in small, controlled movements, keeping the knee bent at 90 degrees and feeling the squeeze in the back of your seat. Keep your abs tight and your hips stacked.

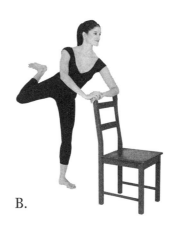

B.

C. Knee to Knee

- Bend your standing (left) knee and turn your right hip toward the floor as you lower your right knee to touch your left knee. Then lift the right leg and hip back up to starting position. Be sure to keep your toes pointed the entire time.

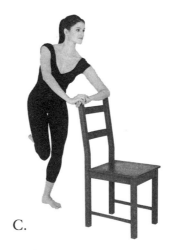

C.

D. Leg Circles

■ Keeping your toes pointed, draw
a circle the size of a tennis ball
with your right knee. Don't twist
your torso while you do this—keep
your rib cage lifting toward the
ceiling.

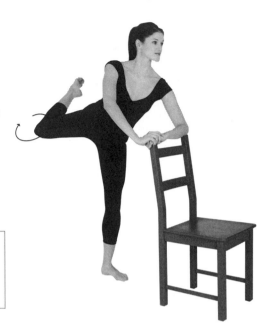

ADVANCED: *Place and squeeze
the ball behind your bent knee
throughout the exercise.*

*Note: When you're first starting out,
or if you have hip issues, it's fine to
keep your working leg lower (but
still out to the side).*

PHYSIQUE 57 TIP

The extent to which you contract
your abs is the extent to which you
will feel your seat muscles working
and changing.

FOLDED L

Our Folded L series takes the concept of weight-bearing exercise to the next level. When you fold your body into an L shape, you rely less on arms and upper body strength and place a deeper focus on your core and standing leg. Don't be concerned if that leg starts to shake—you *will* build your stamina and endurance!

> MUSCLES TARGETED: *Gluteus minimus and maximus, hamstrings, core*
>
> WHAT YOU'LL NEED: *A waist-high, sturdy piece of furniture*

The Setup

- Facing your furniture, place one forearm over the other, leaning forward to let your head rest down on top (this should feel nice for a second!).

- Walk your feet back so that they're right underneath your hips, about hip-width apart—from the side, you should look like a capital letter L.

- Soften both knees and then draw the right heel up toward your right seat muscle (in the workouts, we'll do both sides). Keep your toes pointed and engage your abs. This is your starting position.

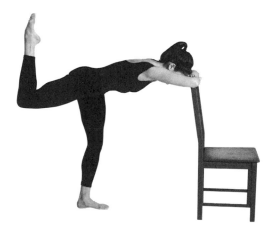

VARIATIONS

A. Pulses Up

■ Keeping your toes pointed, lift and lower your right leg about 2 or 3 inches in small, controlled movements. Concentrate on working from your seat and not letting anything move in your core.

B. Knee to Chest

■ With your toes pointed, bring your right knee in toward your chest and then press it back to the starting position. As you press the leg back, make sure to cinch your abs and keep the spine straight—you want to avoid any arching.

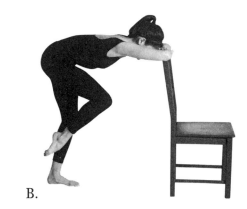

B.

C. Leg Circles

■ Keeping your toes pointed, use your right knee to draw a circle the size of a tennis ball.

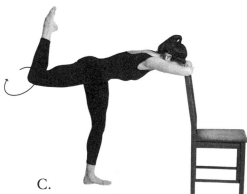

C.

ADVANCED: *Place and squeeze the ball behind your bent knee throughout the exercise.*

Note: *If you have a lower back injury, you can use the Setup posture for Standing Crane (page 91) during this exercise.*

PHYSIQUE 57 TIP

Connect your mind to those areas where you are feeling the burn. When you dig down deep, that's when your body starts to change.

STANDING SCISSOR

We think this one is really hard! But with the biggest challenges come the greatest results. This move combines the power of karate kicks with the grace of ballet's *grand rond de jambe*. Feel your leg reach longer as you stretch to your max, and then watch as you get that sexy, streamlined look from your hips to your toes.

MUSCLES TARGETED: *Gluteus maximus, medius, and minimus; hamstrings; obliques*

WHAT YOU'LL NEED: *A waist-high, sturdy piece of furniture*

The Setup

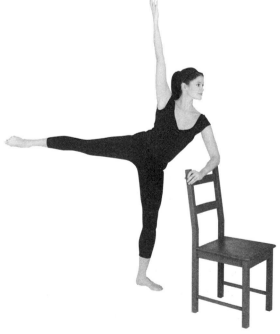

- Stand with your furniture on your left side (in the workouts, we'll do both sides). Lean sideways to place your left forearm on the furniture, keeping your hips in line with your elbow. Now take a big step away from the furniture so that your torso lengthens on an incline.

- Make sure your left foot is directly below your hips (pointing slightly toward your furniture) and soften that knee.

- Raise your right leg up to hip level and straighten it directly out to your side so that your body forms a T shape. Your toes are pointed and your inner thigh is facing the floor.

- Now extend your right arm straight up toward the ceiling. Remember to engage your abs. This is your starting position.

VARIATIONS

. . . .

A. Scissor Movement

- Keeping your toes pointed and your right leg straight, bring the leg forward in front of your chest, keeping your inner thigh facing the floor.

- As you bring the leg forward, slice your right arm down to hip level. The arm stays straight throughout the movement.

- As you bring the leg back to the starting position, your arm goes back up as well.

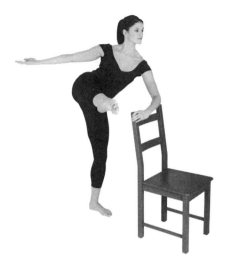

B. Pulse the Leg

- Keeping the right leg straight, bring it forward in front of your chest and put your right hand on your right hip. Your toes should remain pointed.

- With your inner thigh facing the floor, hold the position and pulse the right leg up and down in small, controlled movements, about 2 or 3 inches.

- As you lift and lower, lead with the outside of the leg—this will help you target the outside of your seat down through your outer thigh.

C. Microbends

■ With your right leg still in front of you and your inner thigh facing the floor, bend the right knee slightly and then press it back out, straightening the leg. Your toes remain pointed.

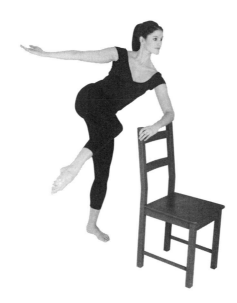

TO MODIFY: *If this is too much at first, you can start with the leg lower or with the knee slightly bent.*

ADVANCED: *Raise the standing heel up so that you're balancing on the ball of your foot for an extra challenge.*

PHYSIQUE 57 TIP

Push your muscles to the point of overload! Make them quiver; make them shake!

PRETZEL

A Physique 57 favorite, the Pretzel is the ultimate multitasking workout move. It simultaneously targets your seat, outer thighs, and waistline to give you a perfectly lifted seat, slimmer thighs, and tightened love handles. Plus, it's gentle enough on your joints that you can do it every day. What more could you ask for?

MUSCLES TARGETED: *Entire seat, abductors, hamstrings, obliques*

The Setup

- Sitting on the floor, bring your left leg in front of you with the left knee bent at a 90-degree angle (in the workouts, we'll do both sides).

- Bring the right leg behind you, and bend that knee at a 90-degree angle as well. Turning your chest slightly left, lean forward and place one hand on each side of your left knee.

- Draw your navel in toward your spine and lift your right leg up off the floor. Point the toes of your right foot and keep them higher than your knee. This is your starting position.

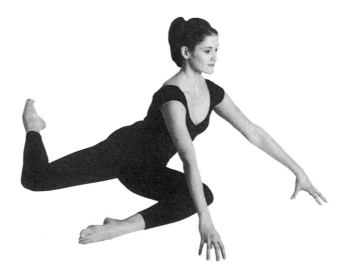

VARIATIONS

. . . .

A. Pulses to the Side

- Keeping your right leg suspended in the air, lift and lower the leg in small, controlled movements using the muscles in the side of your seat. Be sure to keep your toes pointed.

B. Press Leg Back

- Flex your right foot and press your right leg back behind you about 2 to 3 inches in small, controlled movements. Try to keep the ankle above your knee and the heel close to your seat. Make sure your knee stays bent.

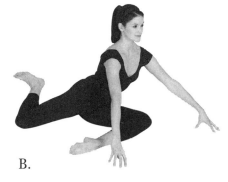

B.

C. Tap Knee, Then Foot

- Keeping your right leg suspended in the air, rotate your right knee to tap the floor, then rotate your right foot to tap the floor. Keep your toes pointed the entire time.

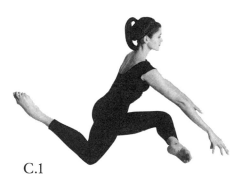

C.1

ADVANCED: *Hold your hands in a prayer position, and/or place and squeeze the ball behind your bent knee throughout the exercise.*

PHYSIQUE *57* TIP

. . . .

Don't be afraid of discomfort in your glutes. If you feel numb at the end of the set, you've done it correctly!

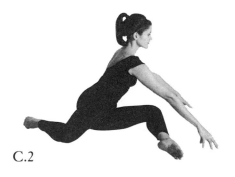

C.2

CLAM

With its laser-like focus directly on the outer seat, the Clam is an awesome way to cinch and smooth the saddlebag area. Break out your pencil skirts!

MUSCLES TARGETED: *Abductors, adductors, obliques*

The Setup

- Lie down on your left side with your left arm extended under your head and your right hand on the floor in front of your chest for support (in the workouts, we'll do both sides). Bend your knees in toward your chest (try to bring them to a 90-degree angle with your upper body).

- Lift your feet off the floor, keeping knees on the floor and your feet together. Keep your shoulders and hips stacked on top of each other, and press your right palm into the floor to engage your obliques.

- Now, keeping your toes together, lift the top right knee above your right hip so that your legs open like a clam. This is your starting position.

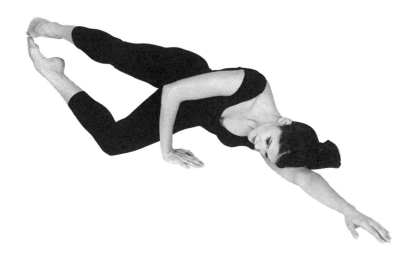

VARIATIONS

A. Pulse Top Knee
- Keeping your toes together, lower and lift the top knee in small, controlled movements, about 2 or 3 inches.

B. Knees Together, Then Apart
- Keeping your toes together, bring your top knee all the way down to the bottom knee and then bring it back up to your starting point.

- As you do this, you may feel your top hip sliding back behind you—don't let it!

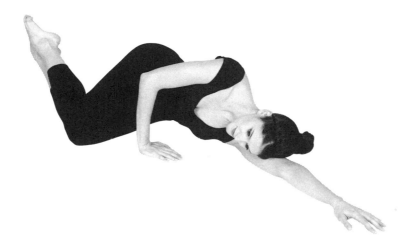

TO MODIFY: *Let the bottom leg rest on the floor for a little bit of extra support.*

PHYSIQUE 57 TIP

When it comes to the seat, the more you squeeze it, the more someone else will want to squeeze it!

HAIRPIN

This one's exactly like the name: A hairpin keeps your hair in place, and this move keeps your seat muscles in place—no bulging, jiggling, or unattractive spread when you sit down. Go for the lifted and perky style!

MUSCLES TARGETED: *Gluteus maximus, medius, and minimus; abductors*

The Setup

- Lie down on the left side of your body and extend your left arm under your head (in the workouts, we'll do both sides). Swing your legs straight in front of you to make a capital letter L. Keep your toes pointed.

- Keeping your hips stacked, press your right palm into the floor in front of your navel to engage your obliques.

- Separate your inner thighs and lift the top right leg so it's in line with your hip. This is your starting position.

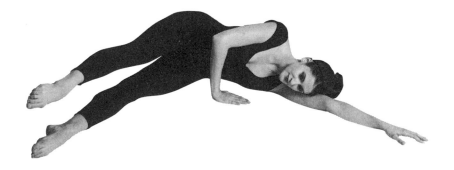

VARIATIONS

A. Pulse the Leg

- Lower and lift your right leg in small, controlled movements, about 2 or 3 inches. As you lift your leg, make sure that you keep your hips and shoulders stacked on top of each other—there's no wiggle room here!

B. Microbends

- Keeping the right leg up, bend the right knee slightly—about 2 or 3 inches—so that your heel comes toward your hamstring, then press it back to the starting position.

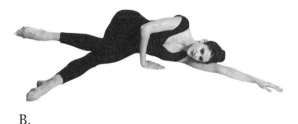

B.

C. Leg Circles

- Keeping your toes pointed, use your right leg to draw a circle the size of a tennis ball.

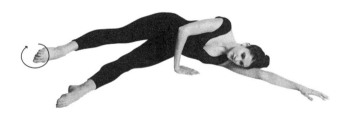

C.

TO MODIFY: *Bend the knee of the bottom leg to give you a little extra support and, more important, keep you in the correct alignment.*

PHYSIQUE 57 TIP

Stay focused on the big picture: If you can get through this, life is easy!

DELI SLICER

Slice off what you don't want hanging off! Women tend to store a lot of fat on the sides of their seat—this move is a fantastic precautionary measure.

> MUSCLES TARGETED: *Gluteus maximus, medius, and minimus; hamstrings; obliques*

The Steps

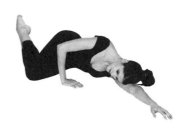

- Lie down on the left side of your body with your left arm extended under your head, and your right palm on the floor in front of your chest for support (in the workouts, we'll do both sides). Bend your knees in toward your chest (try to bring them to a 90-degree angle with your upper body).

- Lift your feet off the floor, keeping your knees on the floor and your feet together. Keep your shoulders and hips stacked on top of each other, and press your right palm into the floor to engage your obliques.

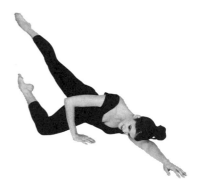

- Now straighten the top right leg, pressing it up and out behind you on a slight diagonal. Then bring it back in. Think of your top knee sliding along the inside of your bottom leg like a deli slicer as you bend and straighten the top leg.

- Make sure you engage your abdominal muscles so that as you push the leg back, you don't arch your back.

> TO MODIFY: *Let the bottom leg stay on the floor for extra support.*

PHYSIQUE 57 TIP

Imagine that you are slicing down cellulite! No lumps or bumps on your bottom!

FIGURE 4 STRETCH

We love this soothing stretch. It feels great in the outer seat muscles, relaxes the neck and shoulders, and gives you time to recharge and refocus between sets—even as it keeps you in the fat-burning zone. After this nice release, you should feel fully recovered and psyched for your next set.

> MUSCLES TARGETED: *Entire seat*

The Steps

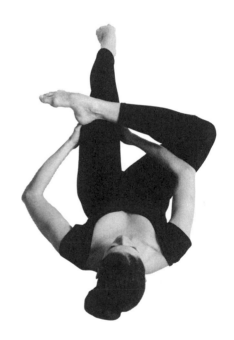

- Lie down on your back with your knees bent and your feet flat on the floor.

- Cross your right ankle over your left knee, and clasp your hands behind your left thigh.

- Pull your left thigh toward your chest and feel the stretch open up your outer right hip and seat area. Keep your spine long and relax your upper back and shoulders.

- Repeat on the other side.

BUTTERFLY STRETCH

This deep hip and seat stretch offers more of an extended recovery. You want to keep your spine long and your hips and tailbone heavy, letting them sink into the floor. Relax for a moment, knowing that after all your Herculean efforts, your body WILL change! So you can enjoy this little break before your Ab series. Ahhhh!

> MUSCLES TARGETED: *Entire seat*

The Steps

■ Lie down on your back with your knees bent and your feet flat on the floor. Cross your right thigh over your left.

■ Lift both legs off the floor, reach for your ankles, and gently pull your legs in toward your chest as far as they will go. Try not to let your heels droop toward your seat. Relax your upper back and shoulders.

■ Switch legs and repeat.

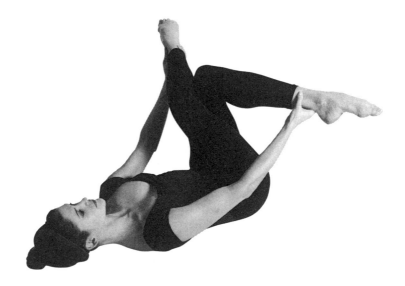

6

ABS

FOR MANY WOMEN, A TAUT, FLAT BELLY IS THE ULTIMATE fitness goal—and it's also one of the hardest to achieve. Contrary to what some diet plans and workouts will tell you, you CAN'T spot-reduce for belly fat. The only way to dramatically shrink or slim down a particular area of the body is to tone the underlying muscles—and in the case of the abs, that means the entire abdominal wall. Your abdominal wall is made up of four distinct muscle groups: the rectus abdominis (what we often call the six-pack); the transversus abdominis, which is the area below the navel; and the internal and external obliques, which lie along the sides of your torso and give shape to your waistline. When sculpted and strong, these muscles work together like a natural corset to pull in your belly and give you a defined, hourglass shape. So if you want to cinch your middle and make that spare tire disappear, you need to strategically target all four sets of muscles—something that traditional sit-ups and crunches fail to do.

Our one-of-a-kind Ab series consists of three different sets of moves done in three different positions: Flat Back, Round Back, and Curl. Together these exercises are able to tighten all four areas of the abdominal wall with equal vigor and precision, and ensure that you activate even hard-to-target areas like the lowermost fibers of the transversus abdominis, or the innermost layers of the obliques. The three sets are differentiated by the degree of spinal flexion: In the first Ab section, we only lift the head and shoulders very slightly to focus on tightening and tucking the area below your navel; in the second, we raise the shoulders up farther to increase the contraction in the abs and involve the muscles of the upper back as well; and in the third, we get the spine moving in all directions—lateral, flexion, and extension—for the deepest contraction yet and to add a burst of cardio for a strong, calorie-burning finish. By changing the position of the spine throughout the three sections, we not only enable you to work the same muscles again and again from different angles, but also protect your neck from the strain that often accompanies ab work. Doing a hundred crunches in a row can tax the neck, especially if the abs are weak—but in our series, we change up the moves every eight to sixteen reps and change the position of the spine every four minutes, ensuring that even as you target your abs with great intensity, you protect yourself from stress and injury.

Throughout these exercises, we will often direct you to lower your legs to your "point of control." Your point of control is the place where your abdominal wall is challenged, and yet you are still able to perform the choreography while maintaining a neutral spine. In neutral spine, there is no excessive arching or tucking, and no excessive tension. If your back starts to arch up off the floor, you've lowered your legs too far. We like working at the point of control because it's the place where you most effectively engage your abdominals: You're achieving the maximum contraction possible without sacrificing form. The two- to three-inch-thick cushion or towel that we use during our Curl section is also intended to help you maintain a neutral spine by supporting the natural curve of your lower back—yet another way that we make sure our abdominal work is always healthy and respectful of your body.

Best of all, you'll find that many of the moves in this chapter will tone far more than just your abs: Our Leg Press move, for example, gives you six-pack abs AND slimmer inner thighs by incorporating the playground ball. We use the playground ball throughout our ab work—sometimes squeezing it between the thighs, sometimes holding it in the hands—to add another layer of isometrics and increase the intensity on the abs. You will also spot several variations that incorporate one of our all-time favorite moves, the Can-Can. We love the Can-Can because its rapidfire movements are one of the fastest ways to generate heat in the body, rev up your caloric burn, and bring you closer to Interval Overload. These dance-type exercises will really get your endorphins going while drawing all the core muscles together and cinching and sculpting them into one long sheath of muscle. Strengthening your core not only does wonders

AB BOOSTERS:

Our Two Favorite Moves for Abs

You can use these moves to supplement your workouts or to tighten up your abs whenever you have a few minutes.

■ Lady Frog: 1 minute (page 116)
■ Showgirl: 1 minute (page 123)

for your waistline, but also helps you stand taller for an overall slimmer look— perfect for when you want to wear that formfitting, sexy dress.

You may notice that our Ab series is the one section of the workout *not* immediately followed by accompanying stretches. This is because we hold back the stretches for the abs until we've finished working the other side of your core: the middle and lower back. So we hit all the muscles of the frontal abdominal wall, then flip over and target the other side with our Back series before stretching the entire core during the Cool Down. In this way, we keep as much heat in your core as possible and ensure that you keep the caloric burn going, rather than releasing the heat and losing momentum as a result.

So let's fire it up! It's time to put on some music and get ready to watch those love handles disappear. This is a meltdown for your waistline! You're going to melt the fat away!

FLAT BACK

Better than any tummy tuck, this sequence of exercises is a fun and highly effective way to target that kangaroo pouch and flatten out your middle. You can literally feel yourself getting tighter with every rep, and as a bonus it stretches your lower back muscles to keep your spine limber and alleviate back pain. Remember that when you're directed to lower your legs, take them just to your point of control—not too low! You want to feel everything in the front of your body contracting toward your spine, NOT feel your spine pulling up off the floor.

> MUSCLES TARGETED: *Entire abdominal wall*
>
> WHAT YOU'LL NEED: *A mat or carpeted floor to lie on; a playground ball*

The Setup

- Lie on the floor with your legs bent, your feet flat on the floor about hip-width apart, your arms resting at your sides. Engage your abdominal wall and keep a neutral spine. This is your starting position.

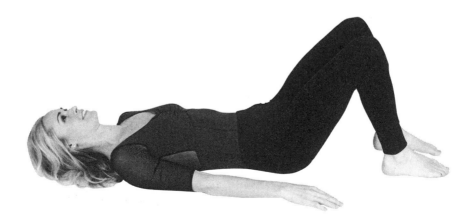

VARIATIONS

A. Bull's-Eye

- Raise your legs and bring them up over your hips. Bend your knees slightly and point your toes.

- Gently lift and lower your hips off the floor. This movement targets the area you *don't* want to call a pouch underneath the navel.

- Do your best to keep the movement strictly vertical—try not to swing your feet forward and back, or side-to-side. Hit your mark on the ceiling like a bull's-eye!

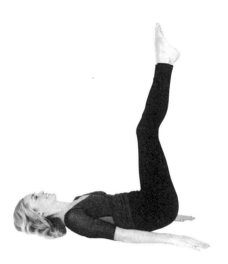

B. Prance

- Bring your knees over your hips. Your feet should be extended out in line with your knees, parallel to the floor, toes pointed. Your arms should float a few inches off the floor, right outside your legs.

- Keeping this shape, curl your head, neck, and shoulders up off the floor as high as you can and begin tapping your toes toward the floor, one foot after the other. Make sure your head and shoulders remain lifted throughout the movement.

- Try to trace the same path with your thighs every time. You'll be whittling down your waistline as you walk!

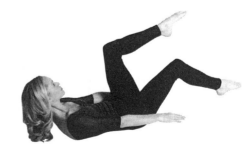

C. Bent Leg Taps

- Bring your knees over your hips. Your feet should be extended out in line with your knees, parallel to the floor, toes pointed.

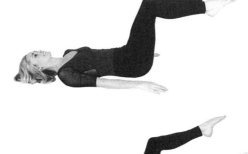

- Keeping your legs bent and glued together, lower your legs to your point of control.

- Now open your legs and then bring them back together to tap them at that point of control. Keep your mind focused on your midline.

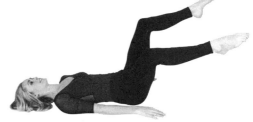

D. Lady Frog

- With your knees over your hips, bring your heels together with flexed feet to form a diamond shape: heels together, toes apart.

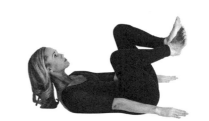

- Curl your head, neck, and shoulders up off the floor as high as you can. Your arms should float a few inches off the floor, right outside your legs.

- Keep your heels together as you straighten your legs and press them out to your point of control. Then bend your knees back in. Make sure that your head and shoulders remain lifted throughout the movement.

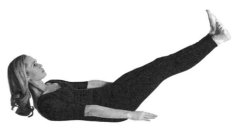

- Every time you press away, draw your navel closer to your spine. Feel everything zipping together! And feel your body getting longer as you stretch all the way from the crown of your head to your heels.

E. Fast Darts with Jabs

- Bring your knees over your hips. Your feet should be extended out in line with your knees, parallel to the floor, toes pointed.

- Curl your head, neck, and shoulders up off the floor as high as you can, and bring your arms into your chest, making a fist with both hands. Your elbows stay close to your sides.

- As you straighten your right leg out toward the floor, twist your torso to the left and jab your right arm past your left knee. Now bend your right leg into your chest, straighten the left leg, and jab your left arm past your right knee. Keep alternating at a good pace, making sure that your head and shoulders remain lifted the entire time.

- You want to straighten your legs as low as you can without letting your lower back arch away from the floor.

- Give a little more energy here—*bring it* with every jab!

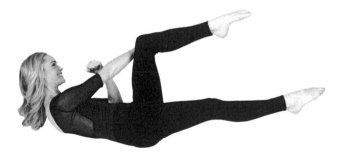

PHYSIQUE 57 TIP

Visualize your perfect waistline! Strong, tucked, no fat on your middle!

F. Bull's-Eye with Ball

- Place the playground ball between your inner thighs, squeezing it just enough to make it form an egg shape.

- Raise your legs and bring them up over your hips. Bend your knees slightly and point your toes.

- Now gently lift and lower your hips off the floor.

- Do your best to keep the movement strictly vertical—try not to swing your feet forward and back, or side-to-side.

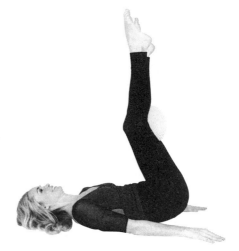

G. Walks with Ball Twists

- Raise your legs and bring them up over your hips. Straighten your legs and point your toes toward the ceiling.

- Lift your head, neck, and shoulders up off the floor as high as you can. With your arms straight, hold the playground ball between your hands above your chest.

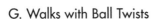

- As you lower your right leg toward the floor, twist your torso to the left, reaching the ball toward the outside of your left ankle. Now bring your right leg back up and lower your left leg while twisting your torso to the right, reaching the ball toward the outside of the right ankle. Continue alternating at a good pace, making sure that your head and shoulders remain lifted the entire time.

H. Leg Press with Ball

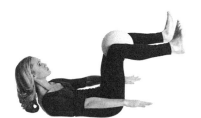

- Bring your knees over your hips. Your feet should be flexed and extended out in line with your knees, parallel to the floor.

- Place the ball between your inner thighs, squeezing it just enough to form an egg shape.

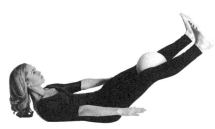

- Curl your head, neck, and shoulders up off the floor as high as you can. Your arms should float a few inches above the floor beside your body.

- Now extend your legs straight away from you at your point of control, then bend them to bring your knees back over your hips. Imagine that you're expanding and contracting your body like a slingshot. Make sure that your head and shoulders remain lifted the entire time.

I. Butterfly Squeezes on the Ball

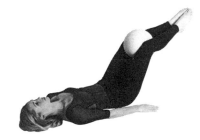

- Raise your legs and bring them up over your hips. Place the playground ball between your thighs and bring your feet together, keeping your toes pointed to make a diamond shape.

- Lower your legs to your point of control, hold them there, and begin performing small squeezes on the ball. Hello, inner thighs!

J. Swirl

- Bring your knees over your hips. Your feet should be extended out in line with your knees, parallel to the floor, toes pointed.

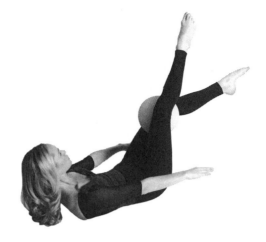

- Place the playground ball between your inner thighs and curl your head, neck, and shoulders up off the floor as high as you can. Your arms should float a few inches off the floor beside your body. Lower your legs to your point of control and hold them there.

- Bring your right leg over your left leg, rotating the ball between your inner thighs. Now bring your left leg over your right leg. Continue rotating at a good pace, making sure that your head and shoulders remain lifted the entire time.

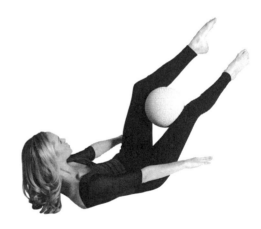

ADVANCED: *Work with your legs straighter and closer to the floor whenever possible. Just make sure you maintain a neutral spine!*

PHYSIQUE 57 TIP

Watch your thoughts—be strong mentally. You'll have more energy if you think of the results.

ROUND BACK

With our Round Back series, you continue to cinch your core while generating a lot of heat and increasing flexibility in the upper and lower back. These dance-inspired ab moves will keep you poised and graceful all day long, with a strong center to boot. Plus, with variations like the Showgirl and the Oblique Can-Can, it's your own personal party—we're so psyched for your midline!

MUSCLES TARGETED: *Entire abdominal wall*

The Setup

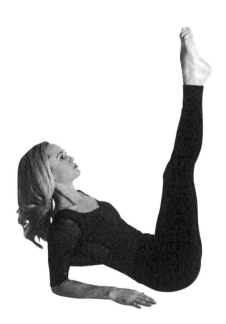

- Lie on the floor and prop yourself up on your forearms with your elbows directly under your shoulders. Your palms are flat on the floor, facing down.

- Raise your legs straight up over your hips, and point your toes toward the ceiling. This is your starting position.

- Try to maintain a concave feeling in your center during these exercises—if you feel like your lower back is starting to arch up off the floor, you've taken your legs too low.

- Try to keep your shoulders away from your ears—imagine even your neck lengthening throughout this exercise.

VARIATIONS

· · · · · · · · · · · · · · · · · ·

A. Single Leg Lift

- ■ Lower your right leg to your point of
  control, then bring it back up to meet
  the left leg (in the workouts, we'll do
  both sides).

- ■ Continue to lift and lower your right
  leg, keeping both legs as straight as
  possible and maintaining a good
  pace.

- ■ As you do this, brace your waistline
  and think about lifting and lengthening
  the right leg rather than just kicking.

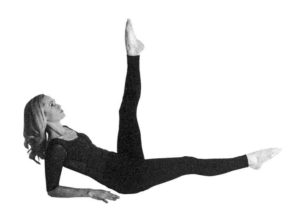

B. Bicycle

- ■ Put the pedal to your middle! Bend
  both knees and start to bicycle your
  legs.

- ■ Aim to draw the biggest possible circle
  you can with your legs—reach all the
  way up to the ceiling and then all the
  way out in front of you.

- ■ Pedal forward first, and then reverse
  your circles.

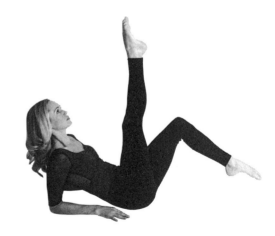

C. Diamond

- Bring your legs into a diamond shape (toes together, knees apart) and lower your legs to your point of control.

- Let your hips feel heavy and sink into the floor; allow your lower back to lengthen.

- Squeeze your knees together and then open back to your starting position. Keep your toes together the entire time.

- Concentrate on initiating the movement from deep within the core. Your inner thighs are working while the abdominals are deeply engaged—get psyched for your newly ripped abs!

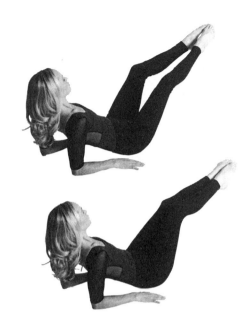

D. Showgirl

- Lower your right leg toward the floor. As the leg goes down, brace your abdominal wall and reach both your arms toward the outside of your left leg.

- As you lift your right leg back up, lower your left leg and twist your torso to reach your arms toward the outside of your right leg. Keep alternating at a good pace.

- Pull in your waistline and imagine yourself onstage—how hard would you pull in that waistline if you were in front of a full house??

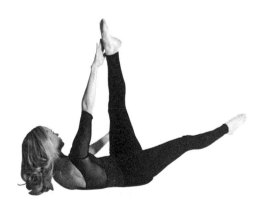

PHYSIQUE 57 TIP

You don't want any belly bulge when you do these exercises—feel that navel, and drive that belly down toward the floor!

E. Oblique Can-Can

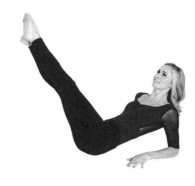

- This is a can-can with a twist—literally! Tilt your legs slightly to the right (in the workouts, we'll do both sides) and then lower them to your point of control. Your left hip should come slightly off the floor.

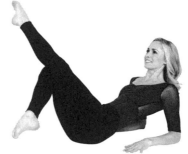

- Keeping your knees together, bend your right leg, bringing the right heel toward your seat. Now straighten the right leg and bend the left leg. Continue kicking one leg at a time, alternating at a good pace. Keep your legs moving as you start to feel the fire in your obliques.

- Stay strong through your core to support your spine—don't let your lower back arch or come up off the floor.

F. Oblique Shuffle

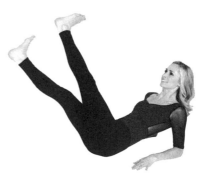

- Tilt your legs slightly to the right (in the workouts, we'll do both sides) and then lower them to your point of control. Flex your feet. Your left hip should come slightly off the floor.

- At your point of control, start to slide your legs past each other in a small, controlled shuffle motion.

- Keep the shuffles small and tight, and make sure you don't feel your lower back starting to move. This variation is great for shedding any signs of unwanted muffin top.

G. Oblique Press-Outs

- Tilt your legs slightly to the right and then lower them to your point of control. Your feet are flexed, and your left hip should come slightly off the floor.

- From there, bend your knees in toward your chest and then press your legs straight out toward your point of control, tracing the same diagonal line every time.

- Think of your body working like a rubber band in this one—as your heels press away, your core contracts deeper to stabilize the movement. Imagine that you're pressing out everything you don't want hanging out!

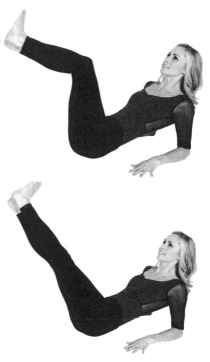

H. Fast Darts

- Bring your knees over your hips. Your feet should be extended out in line with your knees, parallel to the floor, toes pointed.

- Now press one leg at a time straight out, working for maximum extension and control from your core. Continue alternating legs—how fast can you go while keeping your form?

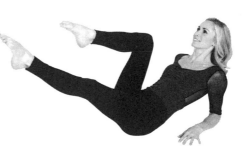

- Be tenacious and bring your biggest energy here—finish this section stronger than you started!

TO MODIFY: *If straight legs are too much, keep your legs bent.*

PHYSIQUE 57 TIP

When you're moving through the reps, don't think, just GO!

CURL

Fierceness now! This is your last chance to attack your abs! Our Curl series is where everything comes together to engage your entire waistline for the ultimate middle meltdown. Your spine is now moving in all directions—lateral, flexion, extension— to target all four sets of abs from every possible angle, and you're squeezing the ball to tap the deepest layers of the abdominal wall. So put on your favorite song and give this section your all. This is where you'll earn your human Spanx!

MUSCLES TARGETED: *Entire abdominal wall*

WHAT YOU'LL NEED: *A 2- to 3-inch-thick cushion or towel; a playground ball*

The Setup

- Sit against the edge of your cushion or towel with your knees bent at 90-degree angles, feet flat on the floor.

- Take your hands to your outer thighs and hold on gently, then roll your torso down until your shoulder blades hover just off the cushion. This is your starting position.

- You want to maintain a concave feeling in your core during all of these exercises—pull your navel in down toward your spine at all times.

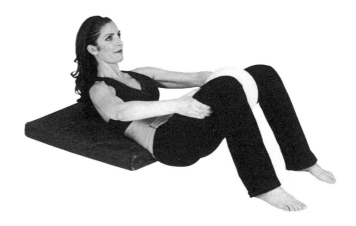

VARIATIONS

A. Curl-Ups with Ball

- Squeezing the ball between your inner thighs, press your feet into the floor. Extend your arms straight along the outsides of your thighs.

- Curl your rib cage up a few inches toward your thighs, and then roll back down to your starting position. These are very small, controlled movements—only about 2 to 3 inches.

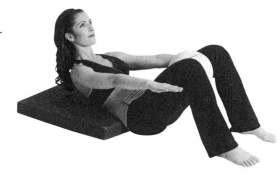

B. Twisted Kickstand

- Squeezing the ball between your inner thighs, extend your right leg straight off the floor (in the workouts, we'll do both sides).

- Twist your torso to the right and begin lifting your rib cage up and down a few inches, reaching your hands toward the outside of the right leg. Try to stay lifted off your right shoulder blade and keep your abs contracted toward your spine. This move is like shrink-wrap for your core!

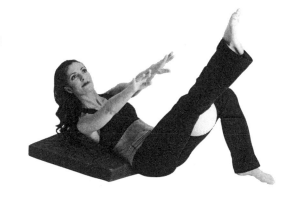

C. Rock-Star Can-Can

- Place the ball between your inner thighs. Extend your right leg straight while simultaneously curling your rib cage up a few inches toward the center. Reach your arms toward your toes.

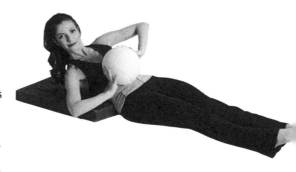

- Now roll back down a few inches as you bend the right leg, and then curl back up again as you extend the left leg. Remember not to roll down too far—your shoulder blades should remain above your cushion the entire time.

- Continue curling and extending at a good pace.

D. Big Twister

- Take the ball between your hands and squeeze it in front of your chest—your elbows should be wide to the side.

- Extend your legs straight along the floor with your toes pointed, keeping your legs together.

- From there, start to twist your upper body from side to side, keeping your shoulders off your cushion, your elbows wide and the ball in front of your chest.

- Make sure you're moving your entire torso here and not just your shoulders—we want to put some fire into your obliques! Twist and shout if you want—we're with you!

PHYSIQUE 57 TIP

Earn your calories! Earn your food!

E. Curl-Ups with Feet on the Ball

- Place the playground ball on the floor. Bend your knees and place your feet on top of the ball, keeping your feet, knees, and thighs together. Your arms should float alongside your thighs.

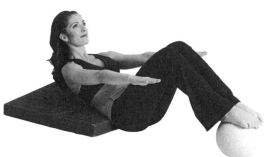

- Curl your rib cage up and down in small, controlled movements, about 2 to 3 inches. Putting your feet on any unstable surface forces you to engage the core muscles at an even deeper level.

F. Superwoman

- Place the playground ball on the floor. Bend your knees and place your feet on top of the ball, keeping your feet, knees, and thighs together. Extend your arms straight out alongside your thighs.

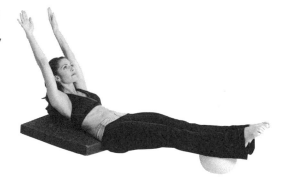

- Now extend your arms up over your head and straighten your legs at the same time, keeping your feet on the ball. The ball will roll out with your feet. Then bring everything back in—you will feel an intense contraction in your core.

- Try not to sit all the way up or fall back onto your shoulder blades as you lower down.

- Go for the gusto! Full extension. Complete contraction. Abs of steel. Do we need to say any more?

G. Shoulder Shimmy

- Extend your legs straight out in front of you with the ball underneath your ankles. Point through your toes.

- Now extend your arms straight out in front of you with your palms facing in.

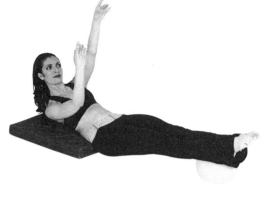

- Pull your navel in, and begin to move your shoulders forward and back, alternating sides so you are "shimmying." As you shimmy, reach through your hands one at a time to lengthen your arms.

- Have your favorite song playing for this one. Dance your way to sexy abs!

H. Rolling Pin

- Bring your feet, knees, and thighs together, and hold the playground ball on your right thigh just below the knee (in the workouts, we'll do both sides). Press your feet into the floor.

- With your hands lightly on top of the ball and your arms straight, curl your rib cage up a few inches toward your right thigh, rolling the ball toward your right knee—you should feel this in your left oblique. Then roll back down to your starting position.

- Envision the rolling-pin effect—as you roll the ball, you're gaining flatness in your abs!

I. Curl-Ups with Ball Press

- With your feet, knees, and thighs together, take the ball between your hands and squeeze it in front of your chest—your elbows should be wide to the side.

- Maintaining the squeeze on the ball, curl your rib cage up and down a few inches in small, controlled movements. Think about hugging your abdominal wall around the ball.

- This fabulous combo briefly shifts the focus to your arms in order to take your mind off your abs. Which do you feel more??

J. Figure 8

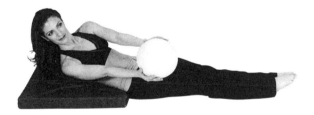

- Extend your legs straight along the floor with your toes pointed, keeping your legs together. Hold the playground ball out in front of your chest with your arms straight.

- Leading with the ball and keeping your arms straight, slowly and deliberately trace a sideways figure 8 in front of you. Make the biggest figure 8 you can. This bonus move will have you feeling both sets of obliques!

TO MODIFY: *Place an extra cushion or towel under your lower back and/or hold on to your outer thighs whenever needed.*

PHYSIQUE 57 TIP

When you do ab work correctly, you should feel your waistline—NOT your neck, lower back, or shoulders.

CHAPTER 7

BACK

WITH ALL THE ATTENTION THAT WE GIVE TO OUR ABS, thighs, and hips on a regular basis, it can be easy to overlook the back. After all, we don't see our back every time we look in the mirror, or worry about whether it looks good in a particular outfit. But strong and supple back muscles are an essential part of the Physique 57 body because they are largely responsible for our posture, helping us to stand taller, look slimmer, and move through the world with grace and ease. Keeping these other core muscles toned and flexible also plays a role in our overall health and wellness by preventing back pain and other back-related issues. Plus, as everyone knows, a sculpted back can be amazingly sexy—why do you think they invented halter tops and backless dresses?

Our Back series focuses on the middle and lower back, and is designed to supplement the upper back and core movements that appear in the Warm-Up and Ab sections. We start off with Back Dancing, which provides a fun way to engage and strengthen your lower back muscles, along with the erector spinae, the two long muscles that run the length of your back and attach to your spine. We also like to think of this exercise as the "last call" for your seat; every time you lift and tuck your hips in this move, you engage the glutes to squeeze those seat muscles one last time.

The second part of our Back series is Back Extensors. For these moves, we lie in a prone position on the floor and then raise our head, arms, and legs to stretch and strengthen the entire back of the body. While most Physique 57 moves make an effort to preserve a neutral spine and prevent excess arching, Back Extensors actually create a deliberate, structured arch that puts a laser-like focus on the lower back muscles and strengthens them in a very safe manner. The moves in this section are reminiscent of Pilates, but we jazz them up by incorporating a playground ball for additional isometrics and stability. With these exercises, all your postural muscles are engaged and you are reaching and lengthening through your spine to produce a strong, flexible, and beautiful back. You'll see the benefits almost immediately as you go about your day standing tall and graceful like a dancer.

At just three minutes long, the Back series is the shortest portion of your workout. But it's also one of the most important, because the gains you make in these three minutes will enhance your health and well-being for years to come. By stretching and strengthening your back and improving your posture and flexibility, you will be able to avoid the back pain and back-related injuries that are incredibly common as we get older. And if you currently experience any pain or discomfort in your lower back, these exercises will do wonders to relieve the pain and restore your muscles and spine to their proper alignment. In fact, the clients who come to us with preexisting back conditions—many of which have persisted for years—often find that after doing our workouts regularly for some time, they no longer need to take pain medication.

So get ready for the final push, and remember that nothing makes you look better than perfect posture! No more slouching, no more hunching—it's time to get tall!

BACK DANCING

This move puts the fun in strengthening your lower back and, as a bonus, it hits the glutes, too. We keep changing your foot position during the choreography so that you feel all the different muscles in your lower back working. By lifting your hips you are also toning your pelvic floor muscles—an easy way to improve your sex life! This is your "Last Call" to work on your bottom, so let's squeeze that seat!

MUSCLES TARGETED: *Erector spinae, seat, lower back*

The Steps

- Lie on your back with your knees bent and your feet parallel, a few inches from your seat and in line with your hips. Your arms rest on the floor at your sides.

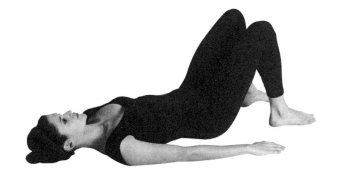

- Now engage your abs and your seat muscles to gently lift your hips up off the floor. With your feet flat, begin performing small, upward tucks with your hips, rolling your tailbone up and then releasing it back. Concentrate on lengthening your spine, not arching it.

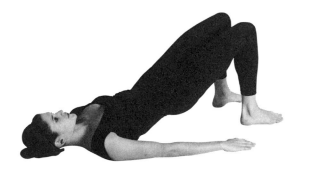

- Now flex your feet so that you are resting on your heels and continue performing hip tucks.

- Now press up onto the balls of your feet—as though you were wearing a pair of high heels— and continue performing hip tucks.

- Concentrate on keeping your rib cage relaxed down toward the floor. You don't want to put the weight into your shoulders.

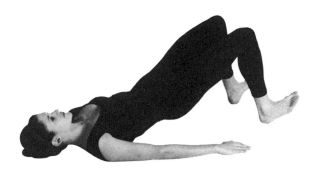

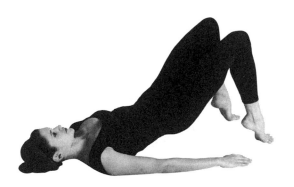

TO MODIFY: *If changing your foot position is too difficult, you can always keep your feet flat for the entire sequence.*

PHYSIQUE 57 TIP

Remember, it's not a competition. Just do the best you can on any given day, and things WILL change.

BACK DANCING WITH BALL

This version of Back Dancing uses a playground ball to challenge your inner thighs along with your glutes and lower back. Toning the lower half of your body was never so much fun!

MUSCLES TARGETED: *Erector spinae, seat, lower back, inner thighs*

WHAT YOU'LL NEED: *A playground ball*

The Steps

- Lie on your back with your knees bent and your feet parallel, a few inches from your seat and in line with your hips. Place the playground ball between your inner thighs and squeeze it just enough to form an egg shape. Your arms rest on the floor at your sides.

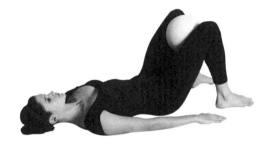

- Now engage your abs and your seat muscles to gently lift your hips up off the floor. With your feet flat, begin performing small, upward tucks with your hips, rolling your tailbone up and then releasing it back.

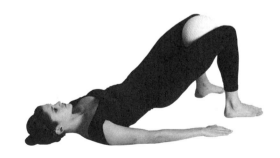

- Now flex your feet so that you are resting on your heels and continue performing hip tucks.

- Now press up onto the balls of your feet—as though you were wearing a pair of high heels—and continue performing hip tucks.

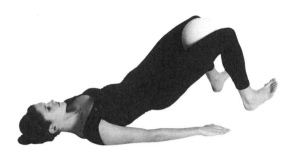

- Concentrate on keeping your rib cage relaxed down toward the floor (you don't want to put the weight into your shoulders).

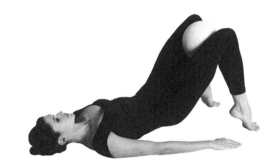

TO MODIFY: *If changing your foot position is too difficult, you can always keep your feet flat for the entire sequence.*

BACK EXTENSORS

No doggy paddling here! It's a full-out sprint now as you swim through your final series of moves. Our Back Extensors strengthen the entire back of your body and engage all your postural muscles for the ultimate finish. Don't slow down now—go for the gold!

> MUSCLES TARGETED: *Entire back*
>
> WHAT YOU'LL NEED: *A mat or carpet under your body; a playground ball*

The Setup

- Lie in a prone position on the floor, extending your arms straight forward and your legs straight back.

- Draw your navel in toward your spine, and then use the muscles in your back to lift your arms and legs off the floor. Your toes are pointed and your head remains in line with your spine so you look down at the floor. This is your starting position.

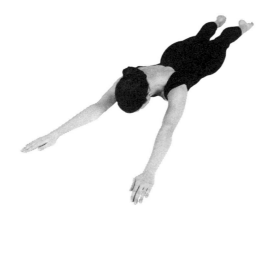

VARIATIONS

· · · · · · · · · · · · · · · · · ·

A. Swimming

- Begin to flutter your legs, kicking in small, controlled movements.

- Now bring your left arm behind you and reach forward with your right arm (in the workouts, we'll do both sides), stretching and lengthening through the entire right side of your body.

- Hold your arms steady while you continue fluttering your legs. Think about reaching longer and lifting up higher. Make sure your head remains in line with your spine.

B. Swimming with Ball

- From your starting position, place the ball under your right hand (in the workouts, we'll do both sides).

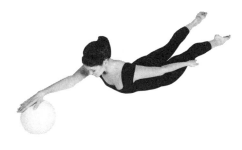

- Now bring your left arm behind you, and continue to reach forward with your right arm, stretching and lengthening the entire right side of the body, and pressing into the ball for support.

- Begin to flutter your legs, as though you were kicking, in small, controlled movements.

C. Mermaid

- From your starting position, bring both arms behind you and clasp your hands together behind your back.

- Keeping your shoulders away from your ears, extend the arms back behind you as far as you can. Make sure that your head remains in line with your spine; do not look up.

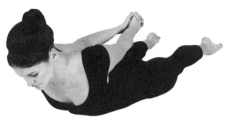

- Keeping your toes pointed and your legs straight, bring your legs in and click your heels together. Continue clicking at a good pace.

D. Mermaid with Ball

- From your starting position, place both hands on top of the ball. Keep your arms extended and your neck in line with your spine.

- Now bring your legs in and click your heels together as you press into the ball for leverage. Keep your toes pointed and continue clicking at a good pace.

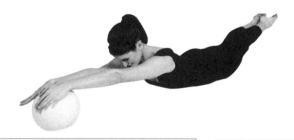

TO MODIFY: *For Swimming, kneel on all fours and reach the opposite arm and leg off the floor at the same time. Then lower the arm and leg and switch sides. Continue alternating at a pace that's comfortable for you, making sure that your neck and spine always remain aligned.*

PHYSIQUE 57 TIP

This is a process and a journey. Every time you do these exercises, you are continuing on the path toward the results you want and a lifetime of good health.

8

COOL DOWN

Mᴇʟᴛ ᴀɴᴅ ʙʀᴇᴀᴛʜᴇ. ʏᴏᴜ'ᴠᴇ ᴇᴀʀɴᴇᴅ ᴛʜᴇsᴇ sᴛʀᴇᴛᴄʜᴇs! Designed to complement all the moves you've just completed, especially those in our Ab and Back series, our three-minute stretch sequence lengthens and relaxes your tired muscles to put the finishing touches on a strong and sexy body. Since you've already been stretching throughout your workout, a few quick moves are all you need to bring your heart rate back to normal, catch your breath, and recharge. Together these six simple stretches release all your muscles and train them to always take their full length, ensuring that you achieve a long, slender, feminine shape.

Whenever you are performing stretches, you want to stretch to the point that you feel a bit uncomfortable, but not push past that spot. Going beyond what your body can handle will *not* make the stretches more effective. So breathe deeply and relax, and remind yourself that your body will become more flexible with every workout. In just two short weeks, you'll be amazed by how much deeper you can go with each stretch, and how much more natural some of these movements feel.

Above all, remember in these moments to congratulate yourself on a job well done! You made it through, and now you can go about the rest of your day knowing that you just did something amazing for your body.

We're so proud of you. Great job, Gorgeous!

CAT/COW STRETCH

Every time you inhale and exhale through this stretch, you create more space between your vertebrae. You'll find that this increased mobility in your spine will help you move more freely throughout your day. You want to move with each breath—let deep inhales and exhales drive these movements.

> MUSCLES TARGETED: *Entire core*

The Steps

- Kneel on all fours, with your hands under your shoulders and your knees directly under your hips.

- Inhale as you round your spine up toward the ceiling, lower your head, and look toward your navel. You want to imagine that someone is gently lifting you up from the middle of your body.

- Now exhale and arch your back, bringing your chin and tailbone up and allowing your navel to sink toward the floor. Drop your shoulders away from your ears so that you feel broad and open through your chest.

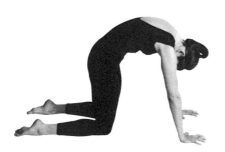 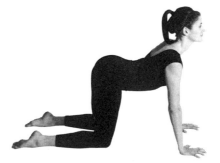

PRONE STRETCH

This stretch returns the natural curve to your lower back. As your shoulders melt down, feel your neck and back muscles release. Take your time with this one—it's okay to stay here a little longer.

> MUSCLES TARGETED: *Anterior spine and abdominal wall*

The Steps

- Lie in a prone position on the floor with your elbows bent and your forearms next to your body.

- Straighten your arms to push your upper body all the way off the floor.

- At the top of the stretch, breathe deeply and release your shoulders away from your ears. Keep your head level and facing forward.

- Bend your elbows and gently lower your upper body back down to the floor.

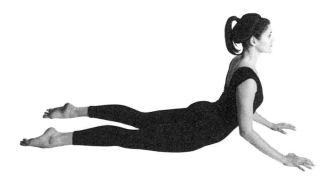

> ADVANCED: *If you need more of a stretch, place your palms directly under your shoulders and press up from there.*

HAMSTRING STRETCH

Tight hamstrings can lead to lower back pain, so take your time here. Remember, it's not about how far you can go into a stretch—go only as far as you can and embrace the sensations you feel now, knowing that your muscles will become more flexible in time.

> MUSCLES TARGETED: *Hamstrings*
>
> WHAT YOU'LL NEED: *A towel (optional)*

The Steps

- Lie on your back and bend your left leg, placing the left foot flat on the floor.

- Extend your right leg up toward the ceiling.

- Place your hands around your calf or ankle (wherever you're comfortable) and gently draw the right leg toward your torso.

- Flex the right foot to press out through your heel—you want to extend the back of your leg as much as you can for maximum benefit.

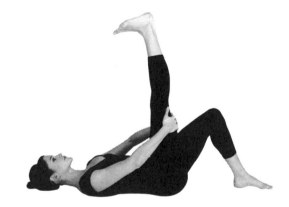

- Repeat on the other side.

> ADVANCED: *If you can keep your pelvis neutral (no arching or tucking), you can extend your left leg on the floor.*

Note: If you can't reach your calf or ankle, don't worry—simply loop a towel or band around the ball of your foot and use it to assist your stretch.

SPINAL TWIST

Allow yourself to wring out any remaining stress or tension! Believe it or not, this soothing stretch is also great for your internal organs.

> MUSCLES TARGETED: *Hips, back, upper body*

The Steps

- Starting in your hamstring stretch, bend your extended right leg in half and place your hands behind your head.

- Gently let your bent leg fall across your body until your knee touches the floor on the opposite side. Allow your right hip to come up off the floor.

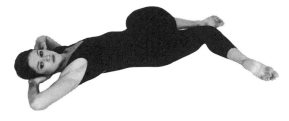

- As you exhale, try to let both your knee and the opposite shoulder drop farther toward the floor so that you can sink deeper into the twist.

- Repeat on the other side.

STRADDLE STRETCH

As you reach the end of your workout, reconnect with your inner dancer. Flow through these stretches with the grace and ease of a ballerina.

MUSCLES TARGETED: *Inner thighs, waistline*

The Steps

- Sit tall on the floor with your legs straight, separating your thighs into a wide V.

- Keep your spine long as you reach your left arm over your head to bend and stretch over your right leg. Try to keep your hips even and the backs of the legs pressing down into the floor. Your chest stays facing forward, and the right arm rests on the floor in front of you.

- Now switch sides and reach your right arm over your head to stretch over your left leg.

- Then walk both arms out in front of you and bend forward at the waist to stretch through the center.

- Play with pointing and flexing your feet to see where you get the maximum stretch.

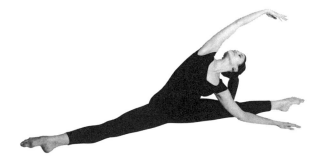

Note: You can also bend one knee and stretch over the extended leg if it's too much to keep them both straight.

FORWARD BEND

Lift your heart up and fold from deep in your hips to melt forward over your legs. Take an extra moment here to acknowledge your accomplishments!

MUSCLES TARGETED: *Hamstrings, back*

WHAT YOU'LL NEED: *A towel (optional)*

The Steps

- Sit tall on the floor with your legs together. They should be extended straight in front of you with your feet pointed.

- Lengthen your spine as you reach both of your arms up to the ceiling.

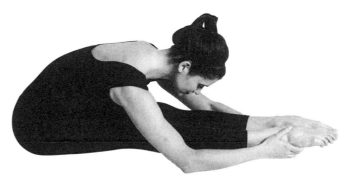

- Now keep the length in your spine as you fold your torso forward as far as possible, leading with your chest.

- When you reach your edge, hold on to your feet or ankles for a breath as you stretch and extend your hamstrings and lower back. Then relax and lift back up.

Note: If you cannot reach your feet or ankles, hold on to your calves, or loop a towel or band around the balls of your feet to assist your stretch.

PART THREE

THE WORKOUTS

NOW THAT YOU'VE LEARNED AND PRACTICED THE moves, it's time to put them together. This section of the book presents the two workouts that are the heart of *The Physique 57 Solution*. Over the next two weeks, you'll be alternating between Classic Workout A (chapter 9) and Classic Workout B (chapter 10) for a total of at least five workouts a week. We've designed the workouts so that they can be performed anytime, anywhere, using only our few standard props and this book. For each workout, we list the moves in their proper order, along with the required number of reps. Just grab your chair and your free weights, cue up your favorite playlist, take a few deep breaths, and you're ready to go!

For each section of the workout, we've also included suggestions about timing—for example, how long the first Thigh section should take, or how much time you should devote to any given stretch. When you're first starting out, don't be concerned if you can't finish a sequence of reps in the exact time allotted. These notes on timing are rough approximations meant to guide you. Do your best to follow them, but don't worry if you run over by an additional thirty seconds or even a minute. We've also taken into account that you will need time to reposition in between sets, so even if you find yourself resting for ten seconds here and there, you should still finish the workout in 57 minutes. That said, again, if you initially run longer, that's okay. It's far more important that you finish the workout and complete as many sets of the reps as you possibly can. As you gain strength and become more comfortable with the moves, you will naturally pick up the pace.

When it comes to performing the moves themselves, bear in mind that some of the series of reps—particularly the longer sets in Seat and Thighs—are going to be very challenging at first. Depending on your level of fitness, you may even find ALL of them very challenging! This is completely normal and even to be expected. So if you can't finish a set, if it's just too hard, it's okay to take a break and then hop back in. Stopping for a few seconds to drink some water and shake out your muscles will ultimately allow you to go further and do more—you can then pick up where you left off and still get the most out of your workout.

You will also most likely experience some soreness in your muscles over the next two weeks as your body adapts to a new level of physical activity. As we've said before, soreness is good because it tells you that your body is changing. Contrary to what most people believe, soreness does *not* mean that you've torn the muscle fibers or injured them in any way; it is simply the body's natural response to an increase in duration and intensity of exercise, and is caused by temporary fluid retention in the muscle fibers. While stretching was long considered the antidote to soreness, recent studies have shown that further physical activity is actually the best way to relieve discomfort. By getting the muscles moving again, you increase blood flow to the area and speed up the adaptation process. So it's fine for you to continue working out, even if you're feeling sore—in fact, we often tell our clients that the very best thing they can do for sore muscles is come back the next day and take another class!

So now it's time to stop talking about the workouts and start DOING them. We're going to kick up your metabolic rate and start creating those long, lean muscles. Before you begin, ask yourself, *Where is my edge today?* And then commit to giving this next workout everything you've got. The next 57 minutes are your time to get strong, and what you put in, you will get back out!

Music to Make You Move: Suggested Playlists

At our studios, we always make an effort to choose upbeat, high-energy music that will keep our clients fired up—even when they're fighting their way through a really killer series of reps. Here are two of our favorite playlists:

Classic Workout A

Warm-Up: "Who Knew" (Bimbo Jones Club Mix), Pink (7:42)

Thigh 1: "4 Minutes" (featuring Justin Timberlake & Timbaland), Madonna (4:05)

Thigh 2: "Calle Ocho 127," Pitbull (5:10)

Thigh Dancing: "Are You Gonna Go My Way," Lenny Kravitz (3:32)

Seat 1: "The Promise," Koishii & Hush (6:08)

Thigh Intermission: "Around the World (La La La La La)," ATC (3:35)

Seat 2: "Band of Gold," Kimberley Locke (6:51)

Ab 1: "SexyBack," Justin Timberlake featuring Timbaland (4:03)

Ab 2: "Down," Jay Sean featuring Lil Wayne (3:53)

Ab 3: "Don't Stop 'Til You Get Enough," Michael Jackson (6:08)

Back Dancing & Back Extensors: "You're the First, the Last, My Everything," Barry White (4:35)

Cool Down: "I Shall Believe," Sheryl Crow (5:34)

Classic Workout B

Warm-Up: "Take a Bow" *(Tony Moran & Warren Riggs Encore Club)*, Rihanna (9:18)

Thigh 1: "Turn Around," Flo Rida (4:00)

Thigh 2: "I Can't Get No Satisfaction," the Rolling Stones (3:45)

Thigh Dancing: "Shake," Ying Yang Twins (4:02)

Seat 1: "Just Can't Get Enough" (12" Mix), Depeche Mode (6:31)

(continued)

Thigh Intermission: "It's Like That," Run-DMC (4:49)

Seat 2: "Alone" (Johnny Budz Extended Mix), Kim Sozzi (6:30)

Ab 1: "Miss You" (Dr. Dre Remix 2002), the Rolling Stones (3:40)

Ab 2: "Dance to the Music," Sly & the Family Stone (4:05)

Ab 3: "Le Freak," Chic (5:32)

Back Dancing & Back Extensors: "Bulletproof," La Roux (3:27)

Cool Down: "Empire State of Mind" (featuring Alicia Keys), Jay-Z (4:37)

9

CLASSIC WORKOUT A

WARM-UP *(approximately 7 to 8 minutes)*

- ■ Knee Lifts—
  60 times, alternating right and left

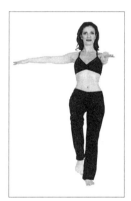

- ■ Biceps Curls—
  60 times, alternating right and left

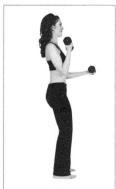

- Shoulder Pulses—
  30 times

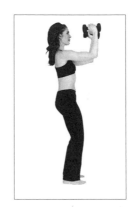

- Rows with Palms In—
  30 times, alternating right and left

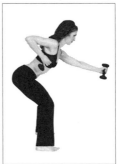

- Triceps Pressbacks (lighter weights)—
  20 times

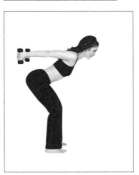

- Push-Ups—
  10 to 15 times

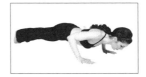

- Plank with Leg Lifts—
  10 each leg

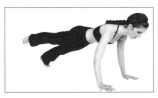

- Forearm Plank with Alternating Knee Bends—20 times, alternating right and left

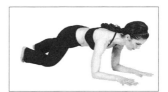

- Triceps Dips— 20 times

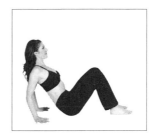

- Triceps Stretch (10 seconds each side)

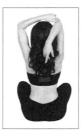

- Shoulder Opener Stretch (10 seconds)

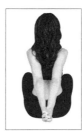

FIRST THIGH SECTION *(approximately 4 minutes)*

- ■ Small V

  - Pulses—8 times

  - Hip Tucks—8 times

  - Seat to Heels and Up—5 to 8 times

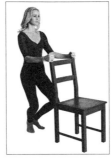

- ■ Small V Incline

  - Pulses—8 times

  - Seat Toward Heels and Up (heels off the floor)—5 to 8 times

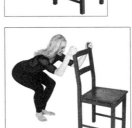

- ■ Small V

  - Hip Shakes right and left (double time!)—8 times each side

  - Hip Circles right and left—4 to the right, 4 to the left

  - Seat to Heels and Up—5 to 8 times

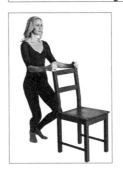

- ■ Small V Incline

  - Pulses—8 times

  - Seat Toward Heels and Up (heels off the floor)—5 to 8 times

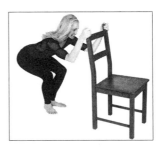

REPEAT entire First Thigh Section 1 more time.

THIGH STRETCHES *(approximately 2 minutes)*

- Standing Quad Stretch (30 seconds each leg)

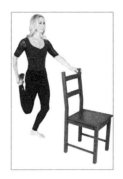

- Hamstring Stretch facing forward
  (30 seconds each leg)

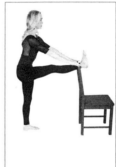

SECOND THIGH SECTION *(approximately 4 minutes)*

- Power Plié with Ball

  - Pulses—8 times

  - Hip Tucks—8 times

  - Hip Shakes—8 times each side

  - Hip Circles—4 to the right, 4 to the left

  - Alternate Heel Raises with Pulses—16 times

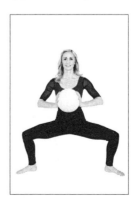

■ Skier with Ball

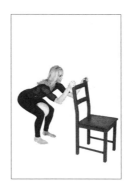

- Squeezes on the Ball—16 times

- Seat Toward Heels and Up
  (heels off the floor)—5 to 8 times

- Squeezes on the Ball—16 times

- Seat Toward Heels and Up
  (heels off the floor)—5 to 8 times

REPEAT entire Second Thigh Section 1 more time.

. . . .

THIGH DANCING *(approximately 1½ minutes)*

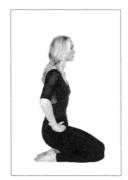

- Hip Tucks—8 times

- Hip Shakes—8 times each side

- Hip Circles—4 to the right, 4 to the left

REPEAT Thigh Dancing sequence 2 more times (3 times total).

. . . .

PUSH-UPS—10 TO 15 *(approximately 30 seconds)*

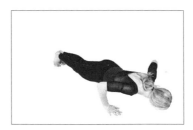

FLOOR STRETCHES *(approximately 2½ minutes)*

- Kneeling Stretch (20 seconds)

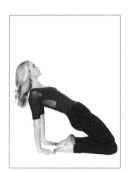

- Gazelle Stretch, right leg forward (30 seconds)

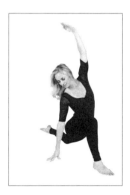

- Anatomically Correct Split, right leg forward (30 seconds)

- Gazelle Stretch, left leg forward (30 seconds)

- Anatomically Correct Split, left leg forward (30 seconds)

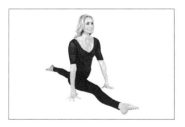

SEAT SECTION,
RIGHT SIDE *(approximately 6 minutes)*

Your right leg is your working leg.

Standing Seat Work *(approximately 3 minutes)*

- Standing Crane

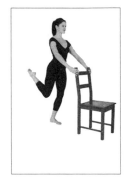

  - Pulses to the Side—8 times

  - Press Leg Back—8 times

  - Speed Skater—8 times

  - Leg Circles—8 to the right, 8 to the left

REPEAT Standing Crane sequence 1 more time.

- Figure Skater

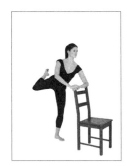

  - Pulses to the Side—8 times

  - Press Leg Back—8 times

  - Knee to Knee—8 times

  - Leg Circles—8 to the right, 8 to the left

REPEAT Figure Skater sequence 1 more time.

Floor Seat Work *(approximately 3 minutes)*

- Pretzel

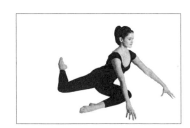

  - Pulses to the Side—8 times

  - Press Leg Back—8 times

  - Tap Knee, Then Foot—16 times

REPEAT Pretzel sequence 1 more time.

■ Clam

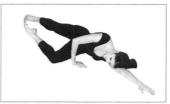

　　• Pulse Top Knee—8 times

　　• Knees Together, Then Apart—8 times

REPEAT Clam sequence 1 more time.

. . . .

FIRST SEAT STRETCH *(approximately 1 minute)*

■ Figure 4 Stretch (30 seconds each leg)

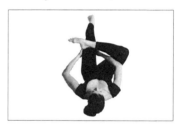

ADVANCED OPTION: *Thigh Intermission (Approximately 1 Minute)*

*Place the playground ball between your inner thighs.

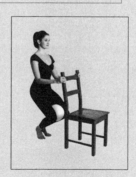

■ Small V with the Playground Ball

　　• Seat to Heels and Up (heels off the floor)—60 seconds

REPEAT entire Seat Section on the
LEFT SIDE *(approximately 6 minutes)*

Your left leg is now your working leg.

SECOND SEAT STRETCH *(approximately 1 minute)*

■ Butterfly Stretch (30 seconds each leg)

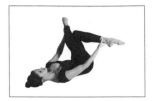

FIRST AB SECTION: FLAT BACK
(approximately 3 to 4 minutes)

■ Bull's-Eye—8 times

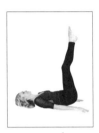

■ Prance (curl head, neck, and shoulders up)—16 times, alternating right and left

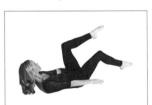

■ Bent Leg Taps—16 times

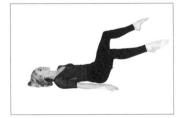

■ Lady Frog (curl head, neck, and shoulders up)—8 times

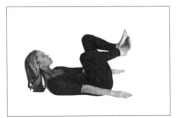

- Fast Darts with Jabs (curl head, neck, and shoulders up)—16 times, alternating right and left

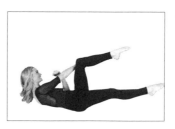

REPEAT Flat Back sequence 2 more times (3 times total).

TRICEPS DIPS—20 TIMES *(approximately 30 seconds)*

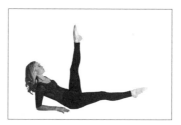

SECOND AB SECTION: ROUND BACK

(approximately 3 to 4 minutes)

- Single Leg Lift—4 times right, 4 times left

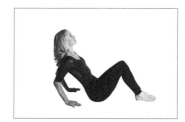

- Bicycle—8 forward, 8 backward

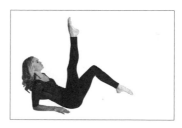

- Diamond (squeeze knees together and apart)—16 times

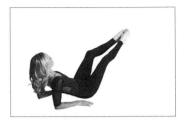

- Showgirl—16 times, alternating right and left

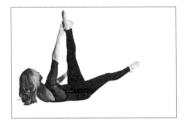

REPEAT Round Back sequence 2 more times (3 times total).

FOREARM PLANK *(approximately 20 seconds)*

- Hip Twists—10 times each side

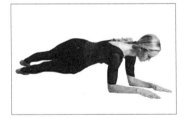

THIRD AB SECTION: CURL

(approximately 4 to 5 minutes)

*Place the playground ball between your inner thighs.
- Curl-Ups with Ball—16 times

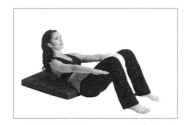

- Twisted Kickstand over right leg—16 pulses
- Twisted Kickstand over left leg—
  16 pulses

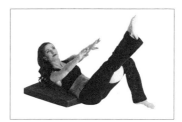

- Rock-Star Can-Can (can-can legs with curl-ups)—16 times, alternating right and left leg

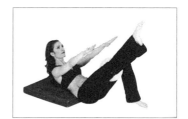

REPEAT Curl sequence 2 more times (3 times total)—
you can rest 10 seconds and reset the position in between sets.

*Hold the ball in your hands in front of your chest.
- Big Twister (legs straight on the floor, tap the ball right and left)—15 taps each side

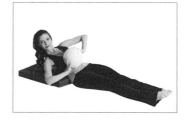

BACK DANCING *(approximately 2 minutes)*

Feet parallel, hip-width apart
- Hip Tucks

  - Feet flat—16 tucks

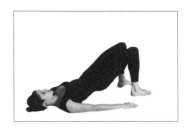

  - Feet flexed—16 tucks

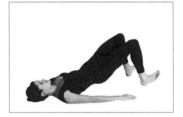

  - High heels—16 tucks

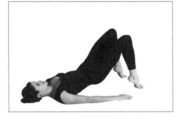

REPEAT Back Dancing sequence 2 more times (3 times total).

BACK EXTENSORS *(approximately 1 minute)*

- Swimming with right arm back—8 times
- Swimming with left arm back—8 times

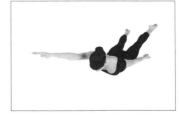

- Mermaid—16 clicks

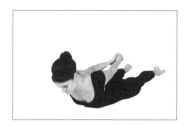

REPEAT Back Extensors sequence 1 more time.

COOL DOWN *(approximately 3 minutes)*

- Cat/Cow Stretch—2 times

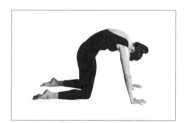

- Prone Stretch—20 seconds

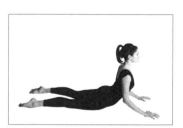

- Hamstring Stretch—10 seconds each side

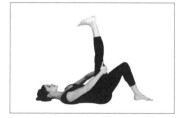

- Spinal Twist—10 seconds each side

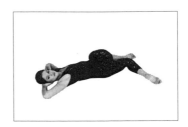

- Straddle Stretch—10 seconds each to right, left, and center

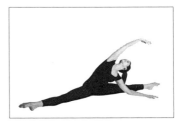

- Forward Bend—20 seconds

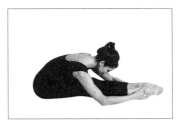

10
CLASSIC WORKOUT B

WARM-UP *(approximately 7 to 8 minutes)*

- Knee Lifts—60 times, alternating right and left

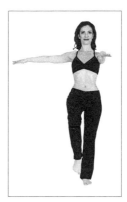

- Hammer Curls—30 times, alternating right and left

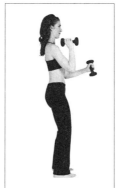

- Shoulder Pulses—30 times

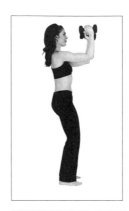

- Rows with Wide Elbows—30 times,
  alternating right and left

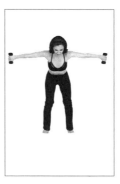

- Scarecrows (lighter weights)—20 times

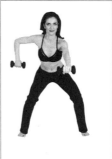

- Triceps Pressbacks
  (lighter weights)—20 times

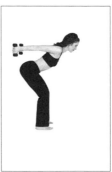

- Push-Ups—10 to 15 times

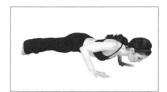

- Plank with Leg Lifts—10 each leg

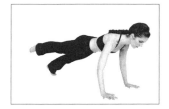

- Forearm Plank with Both Knees Bending—20 times

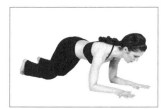

- Triceps Can-Can—10 times each leg

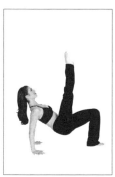

- Triceps Stretch—(10 seconds each side)

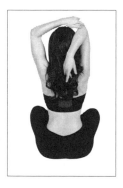

■ Shoulder Opener Stretch—10 seconds

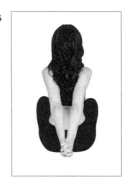

FIRST THIGH SECTION *(approximately 4 minutes)*

■ Swivel Chair right

- Pulses—8 times

- Hip Tucks forward—8 times

- Seat to Heels and Up—5 to 8 times

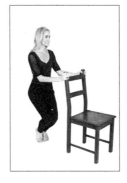

■ Skier (feet flat, incline spine forward)

- Pulses—8 times

- Seat Toward Heels and Up (heels off the floor)—5 to 8 times

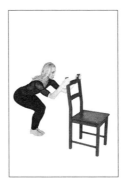

- Swivel Chair left

  - Pulses—8 times

  - Hip Tucks forward—8 times

  - Seat to Heels and Up—5 to 8 times

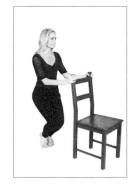

- Skier (feet flat, incline spine forward)

  - Pulses—8 times

  - Seat Toward Heels and Up (heels off the floor)—5 to 8 times

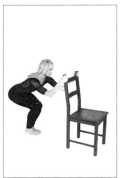

REPEAT entire First Thigh Section 1 more time.

THIGH STRETCHES (approximately 2 minutes)

- Standing Quad Stretch (30 seconds each leg)

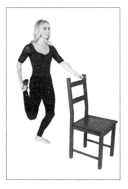

- Hamstring Stretch facing forward
  (30 seconds each leg)

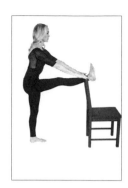

SECOND THIGH SECTION

(approximately 4 minutes)

- Curtsy with right leg back

  - Pulses—16 times

  - Single Leg Pulse (right leg off the
    floor)—16 times

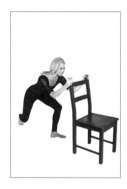

- Small V

  - Seat to Heels and Up—5 to 8 times

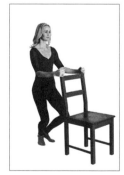

- Curtsy with left leg back

  - Pulses—16 times

  - Single Leg Pulse (left leg off the floor)—16 times

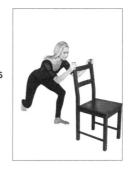

- Small V

  - Seat to Heels and Up—5 to 8 times

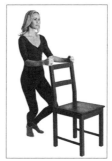

REPEAT entire Second Thigh Section 1 more time.

. . . .

THIGH DANCING WITH BALL

(approximately 1½ minutes)

*Squeeze the ball between your inner thighs.
- Pulses Off Heels—8 times

- Hand Jive—8 times

- Boxer Girl (arm jabs with hip shakes—double time!)—16 times

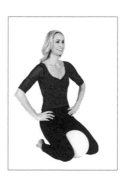

REPEAT Thigh Dancing sequence 2 more times (3 times total).

FOREARM PLANK WITH BALL *(30 seconds)*

- Both knees bending with ball—20 times

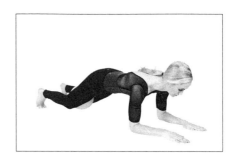

FLOOR STRETCHES *(approximately 2 minutes)*

- Kneeling Stretch (20 seconds)

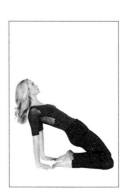

- Gazelle Stretch, right leg forward (30 seconds)

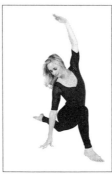

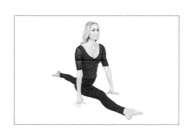

- Anatomically Correct Split, right leg forward (30 seconds)

- Gazelle Stretch, left leg forward (30 seconds)

- Anatomically Correct Split, left leg forward (30 seconds)

SEAT SECTION, RIGHT SIDE

(approximately 6 minutes)

*Your right leg is your working leg.

Standing Seat Work *(approximately 3 minutes)*

- Folded L

  - Pulses Up—8 times

  - Knee to Chest and press back up—8 times

  - Leg Circles—8 to the right, 8 to the left

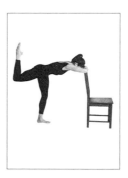

REPEAT Folded L sequence 1 more time.

- Standing Scissor

  - Scissor Movement—8 times

  - Pulse the Leg—8 times

  - Microbends—16 times

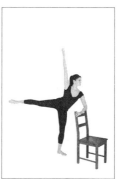

REPEAT Standing Scissor sequence 1 more time.

Floor Seat Work (approximately 3 minutes)

- Hairpin

  - Pulse the Leg—8 times

  - Microbends—16 times

  - Leg Circles—4 to the right, 4 to the left

  - Deli Slicer—16 times

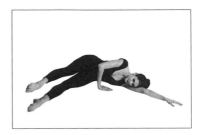

REPEAT Hairpin sequence 1 more time.

....

FIRST SEAT STRETCH *(approximately 1 minute)*

- Figure 4 Stretch (30 seconds each leg)

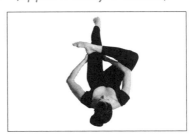

ADVANCED OPTION: *Thigh Intermission (Approximately 1 Minute)*

- Kick Line

  - Pulses with pointed toes—8 times

  - Grande Battement—8 times

  - Microbend with Flexed Foot—16 times

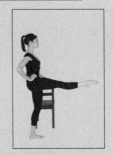

REPEAT Kick Line sequence 1 more time, and then switch to the other leg and do 2 sets.

REPEAT entire Seat Section on the LEFT SIDE *(approximately 6 minutes).*
Your left leg is now your working leg.

SECOND SEAT STRETCH *(approximately 1 minute)*

- Butterfly Stretch (30 seconds each leg)

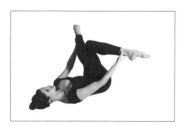

. . . .

FIRST AB SECTION: FLAT BACK WITH BALL *(approximately 3 to 4 minutes)*

Place the playground ball between your inner thighs.
- Bull's-Eye with Ball (pointed toes)—8 times

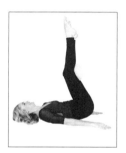

- Leg Press with Ball (curl head, neck, and shoulders up)—8 times

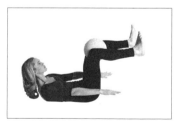

- Butterfly Squeezes on the Ball (with toes together)—16 times

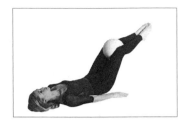

- Swirl (curl head, neck, and shoulders up)—8 times, alternating right leg over, then left leg over

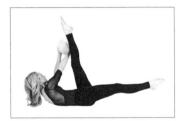

- Walks with Ball Twists (curl head, neck, and shoulders up)—8 times each side, twisting right, then left

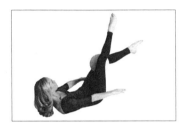

REPEAT Flat Back sequence 2 more times
(3 times total).

TRICEPS DIPS—20 TIMES *(approximately 30 seconds)*

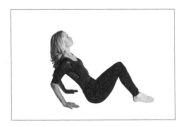

SECOND AB SECTION: ROUND BACK

(approximately 3 to 4 minutes)

Swing legs to the right; lower to your point of control.

- ■ Oblique Can-Can—8 times, alternating right then left

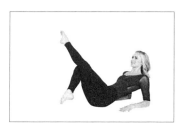

- ■ Oblique Shuffle—16 times, alternating right then left

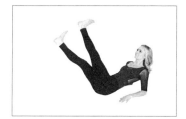

- ■ Oblique Press-Outs—8 times

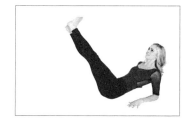

Center—bend your knees at a 90-degree angle.

- ■ Fast Darts—16 times, alternating right then left

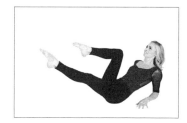

Swing legs to the left; lower to your point of control.

- ■ Oblique Can-Can—8 times, alternating right then left

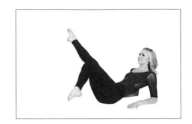

- ■ Oblique Shuffle—16 times, alternating right then left

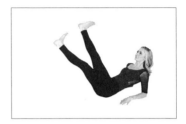

- ■ Oblique Press-Outs—8 times

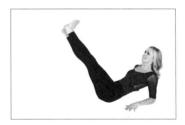

Center—bend your knees at a 90-degree angle.

- ■ Fast Darts—16 times, alternating right then left

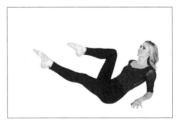

REPEAT Round Back sequence 1 more time.

FOREARM PLANK *(approximately 30 seconds)*

- Hip Twists—10 times each side

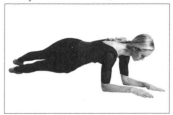

··

THIRD AB SECTION: CURL WITH BALL
(approximately 4 to 5 minutes)

Feet on the ball, legs bent
- Curl-Ups with Feet on the Ball—8 times

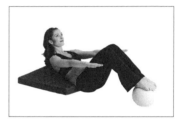

- Superwoman (extend arms and legs straight, then pull back into chest)—8 times

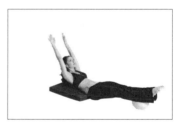

- Shoulder Shimmy (legs straight on the ball)— 16 times, alternating right shoulder, then left shoulder

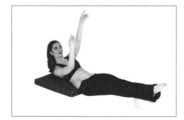

REPEAT Curl sequence 2 more times (3 times total)—can rest 10 seconds and reset position in between sets.

Take the ball in your hands and bring your knees, thighs, and feet together.

■ Rolling Pin (roll ball up bent legs)

• Roll ball up the right thigh—8 times

• Roll ball up the left thigh—8 times

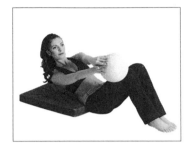

■ Curl-Ups with Ball Press (ball between hands at chest)—8 times

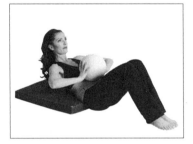

REPEAT Rolling-Pin/Curl-Ups sequence 2 more times (3 times total).

Straight legs

■ Figure 8 with ball—30 times

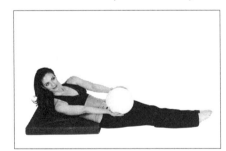

BACK DANCING WITH BALL

(approximately 2 minutes)

Place the ball between your inner thighs.

■ Hip Tucks

    ● Feet flat—16 tucks

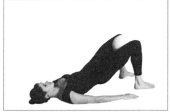

    ● Feet flexed—16 tucks

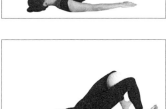

    ● High heels—16 tucks

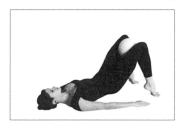

REPEAT Back Dancing sequence 2 more times (3 times total).

BACK EXTENSORS WITH BALL
(approximately 1 minute)

- Swimming with right arm back, left hand on ball—8 times

- Swimming with left arm back, right hand on ball—8 times

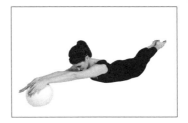

- Mermaid with ball—16 clicks

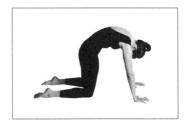

REPEAT Back Extensors sequence 1 more time.

. . . .

COOL DOWN *(approximately 5 minutes)*

- Cat/Cow Stretch—2 times

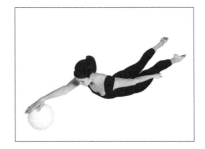

- Prone Stretch—20 seconds

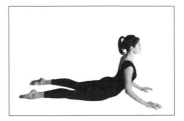

- Hamstring Stretch—10 seconds each side

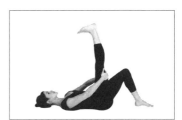

- Spinal Twist—10 seconds each side

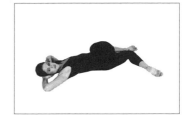

- Straddle Stretch—10 seconds each to the right, left, and center

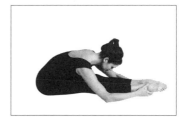

- Forward Bend—20 seconds

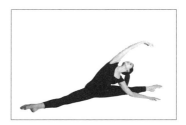

PART FOUR

THE MENU

11

EAT, DRINK, AND BE GORGEOUS

PHYSIQUE 57 HAS NEVER BEEN ABOUT BEING SUPER-skinny. It's about gaining strength, building muscle, and feeling great in the body that you've been given. But for many of us, getting fit also means shedding the excess pounds we may have been carrying around, sometimes for years. The Physique 57 meal plan is a delicious, all-natural, macronutrient-rich approach to weight loss designed to complement our workouts and melt away the pounds. Whether you're looking to lose five pounds or fifty, our recipes will help you cut calories, rev up your metabolism, and shed "false fat"—the water weight, bloating, and inflammation that result from eating certain types of foods. Our tasty dishes will also fortify your body so that you get the most out of your workouts by boosting your energy, giving you plenty of lean protein, and providing you with a hefty dose of vitamins and nutrients that will jump-start your body's own natural weight-loss process.

Our plan starts by cutting out all of the foods that potentially stress your body: processed and denatured foods, allergenic foods such as wheat and soy, and foods loaded with synthetic additives and preservatives. We then replace them with "powerhouse" foods that deliver a big nutritional punch: high-quality protein, organic fresh fruits and vegetables, organic whole grains, and healthy fats. Most people today eat far too many processed foods because they're inexpensive and easy to prepare. Too often we fall back on frozen dinners, energy drinks, or vending-machine fare to get us through the day. Unfortunately, these foods tend to be loaded with chemicals and synthetic ingredients that are toxic to the body and cause swelling and inflammation that can persist in the form of excess pounds. This toxicity also slows your body's metabolism, making it harder for you to burn calories efficiently, and leaving you feeling tired and lethargic. To top it off, these unhealthy foods cause you to eat more than you really need, due to their shockingly low nutritional value. If you eat empty calories, you're not going to feel full or satisfied, and your body will continue to crave more and more food as it tries to acquire the vitamins and nutrients it needs. By taking unhealthy foods out of your diet and adding those that fuel your system in a healthy way, you are giving your body what it needs to function properly and do what it's designed to do—achieve your optimum weight.

Many processed and allergenic foods are also high in fats and sugars, so when we eliminate them entirely, cutting calories becomes a snap. Soon it's incredibly easy to stay within an ideal range of fourteen hundred to sixteen hundred calories a day. Numerous studies have shown that in order to lose weight at a steady, significant rate—*without* also losing lean body mass—you want to generate a deficit of approximately five hundred calories per day. And if you combine our daily meal plans with our high-intensity workouts, that is exactly what you will achieve. The good news is that we've done all the guesswork for you so that you don't have to spend time counting calories or tracking points. All you need to do is follow our recipes and guidelines, and you will automatically reduce your caloric intake and find that sweet spot where the pounds are coming off, even as you are gaining muscle.

But the very best part of our two-week plan is that eating this way is actually a pleasure. We've done our best to give you foods that you are going to LOVE, whether you're looking to lose weight or just seeking a healthier lifestyle. You will be amazed to discover how delicious and satisfying simple dishes like Herbed Salmon or Baked Apples can be, or how tasty a low-calorie, low-fat dish like our Easy "Tortilla" Soup can be for lunch. Each recipe is packed with flavor as well as nutrients, and we give you plenty of tips and options to customize the dishes to your own particular tastes and preferences. Above all, we promise that you won't go hungry—these dishes are yummy and substantial enough to fill you up. And for the moments when you need a pick-me-up or a quick burst of energy to fuel your workouts, we've provided a list of healthy snacks and munchies that you can reach for throughout the day.

You will likely find that after only a few days on our meal plan, your energy will skyrocket and your cravings for sweets and junk food will begin to disappear. You will also begin to notice changes in your complexion—even your skin will have that proverbial "glow." Eating right affects far more than just your weight, and many of our clients feel so good on our program that they continue to eat this way long after the first two weeks are up. We hope that you will want to follow in their footsteps and use our recipes to look and feel gorgeous for the rest of your life.

Here are five simple steps to get you started.

Step 1: Cut Out the Junk

For these two weeks, we want you to be especially strict about avoiding junk and the chemicals found in processed foods. Your new rule of thumb, with minimal exceptions, should be: *If it doesn't occur in nature, don't eat it!* We also ask you to eliminate the most allergenic foods—such as milk, wheat, corn, and soy—because even if you don't have an identified food allergy, they can still cause inflammation in the body.

Your new eating guidelines are:

- NO processed foods. This means anything packaged or modified by people other than you. Most of these foods will be found in the center aisles of your grocery store, and you will be shopping from the outer sections with the fresh fruits, vegetables, and meats instead. We do make a few exceptions for some of the seasonings in our recipes, such as tamari, hot sauce, and vanilla extract, and several of our snack options, including organic gluten-free crackers, and canned wild salmon and sardines. As long as you buy these items organic, you'll be fine.

■ NO wheat. This may be challenging for those who love their carbs, but wheat is a major allergen, and most of the wheat in the United States is genetically engineered—it contains very few natural nutrients and little fiber. Fortunately, there are a variety of healthy grains that you can substitute, such as brown rice, oats, and quinoa.

■ NO sugar, except what occurs naturally in fruits, vegetables, and other whole foods. Processed sugar, which started off as a lush, green plant, has been stripped of all fiber and nutritional value. Eating too much will spike your insulin levels, taxing your pancreas and putting you on the road to diabetes. And when your insulin levels spike, your body releases stress hormones that in turn cause inflammation and false fat. On our plan, we enjoy natural, unprocessed sugars that come with a cushion of fiber and nutrients, such as raw honey, grade B maple syrup, and the sugars (or fructose) found in fruits, which feature prominently in our desserts.

■ NO corn. This includes the high-fructose corn syrup found in many processed foods. Corn is highly allergenic, and most of the corn products commercially available today are genetically modified.

■ NO soy. Not only is soy a major allergen, but it also contains other components, such as phytoestrogens, that can be stressful to your system. Asian cultures ferment their soy, which changes its composition and makes it easier for your body to process. The only permissible soy on our program is organic tamari (wheat-free soy sauce), which has been properly fermented and is easier for your body to digest. If you are a vegetarian, we do allow you to substitute tofu and tempeh for the animal protein in some of our dishes—just be sure you follow the guidelines for using these foods on page 201.

■ NO milk. Milk is a source of highly concentrated calories meant to nourish a baby calf, an animal that nature designed to grow from fifty pounds to two thousand in just six months! If you're trying to lose weight, you want to stay away from milk and most dairy products. In addition, the synthetic hormones and antibiotics found in non-organic dairy can stress your body and create swelling.

- NO low-fat or sugar-free foods. These foods have been modified from their original state and may contain chemicals or additives as a result.
- NO artificial sweeteners. Anytime you eat something that your body doesn't recognize, it creates toxicity, which keeps the weight on.
- NO iodized salt. This means processed salt, which is artificially enriched with synthetic iodine, contains chemicals, and lacks the fifty trace minerals found in sea salt. By substituting sea salt, you will get not only naturally occurring iodine but plenty of additional nutrients that your body needs.
- NO alcohol. For your purposes during these two weeks, all alcohol, even wine, is a source of empty calories. You don't need it! Some kinds of alcohol, such as beer, are derived from grains and allergenic wheat.

If you follow our recipes, you will avoid these foods automatically, but do your best to keep these guidelines in mind whenever you eat out or need to grab food on the go.

CALORIE CULPRITS: THE BIGGEST SOURCES OF HIDDEN CALORIES

Even after the first two weeks are up, you'll do well to avoid these calorie-packed and sugar-laden foods if you want to keep your newly slim and sexy physique:

- Alcoholic beverages. Cocktails, especially sweet ones, are chock-full of calories. A martini has 200 calories, a cosmopolitan has 213, and a margarita has a whopping 540 calories. Beer has an average of around 150, but if you have more than one, the calories can add up quickly. Worst of all, these empty calories won't even satisfy your hunger—instead, they will cause your blood sugar to spike and then crash, leading to a craving for food and sweets.
- Vitamin drinks, sports drinks, and energy drinks. Believe it or not, "enhanced" water sometimes isn't water at all—it can actually contain more than a hundred calories! And sports and energy drinks contain anywhere from 160 to 310 calories. Plus, these drinks are loaded with the chemical additives and

(continued)

high-fructose corn syrup that lead to false fat. For a refreshing alternative, try our Citrus Cooler on page 272.

■ The bread basket at restaurants. This is a total waste of calories. If you skip the bread basket when eating out, you will automatically reduce your caloric intake by anywhere from 170 to 300 calories.

■ Passed hors d'oeuvres at parties. These generally have 70 to 110 calories each— and they are bite-size!

■ Granola. This is always touted as a health food, but in reality, a quarter-cup-size portion has 250 calories…and no one eats just a quarter cup!

■ Smoothies from franchised smoothie stores. The base for these smoothies has a ton of sugar—you'll do better to make one of our smoothies on page 274.

■ Pasta. Pasta is technically a fat-free food, but a serving is considered to be only half a cup—and most restaurants will give you three or four cups! By the time you add the sauce, you're looking at a twelve-hundred-calorie commitment for a single dish.

■ Salads and salad bars at restaurants. You never know what they're using to make the dressings or prepare the protein toppings. One Chinese Chicken Salad at a popular chain restaurant contains thirteen hundred calories! To make the salad bar work for you, do a once-around to check out the offerings and choose what you recognize as real/whole foods—the less cooked or processed, the better. Then make your own simple dressing with olive oil, vinegar, and a squeeze of lemon. When ordering a salad in a restaurant, always ask for the dressing on the side.

■ Foods marked FAT FREE. Fat-free foods can be particularly bad calorie-wise—they may be low in fat but high in sugar. Jelly beans are touted as a fat-free food, for instance, but they will still pack on the pounds.

Step 2: Eat Macronutrient-Rich Foods in the Proper Portions

The word *macronutrient* refers to the three essential nutrients found in food that your body needs for energy and a host of other functions: proteins, carbohydrates, and fats. These macronutrients play a vital role in every system in the body: They give us energy, help us build lean muscle, and regulate metabolism and hormone production. The quality of the macronutrients you ingest plays an enormous role in how you look and how well your body functions. When it comes to gaining or losing weight, these macronutrients influence everything from your metabolic rate to how quickly you are able to build and preserve lean muscle. They also help you to process and absorb key vitamins and minerals, and manufacture others, such as vitamin A, that aren't found in nature. When we overprocess or refine foods, or change a food's composition by making it low-fat or by adding chemicals or preservatives, we end up altering or stripping away many of the macronutrients that greatly enhance our overall health.

For the next two weeks, we want to fuel your body for optimum energy and performance, so our goal is to provide you with high-quality foods that offer heaping doses of macronutrients in their purest form. This means that we focus on whole or unrefined foods: fruits, vegetables, greens, and lean protein, with small amounts of grains and dairy. With every spoonful of food, we want you to get as many nutrients, vitamins, and minerals as you possibly can.

Here's what you will find on our menus:

Lean Protein
Two to three servings a day, plus one snack if needed.
1 serving = 4 to 6 ounces or ¾ cup.

Proteins are the building blocks of every cell, tissue, and organ in your body, and they are essential for a host of bodily functions, including two that are especially important while you're on this program: regulating metabolism and preserving lean muscle. Protein is made up of smaller units called amino acids, but only certain kinds of animal protein contain all twenty of the essential amino acids that your body needs. Our plan focuses on:

- Free-range eggs, chicken, and turkey that have been raised without the use of growth hormones or antibiotics.
- Grass-fed lamb and beef that are also hormone- and antibiotic-free.
- Healthy fish such as wild salmon, tilapia, sole, flounder, sardines, and anchovies that have the lowest levels of mercury and other contaminants.

By choosing these high-quality proteins, you will not only avoid the synthetic chemicals and hormones that can cause inflammation and false fat, but also receive more vitamins and nutrients overall. Compared with regular red meat, grass-fed beef and lamb, for example, contain much higher levels of vitamin D and omega-3 fatty acids, which reduce inflammation and LDL—or "bad"—cholesterol, and act as carriers for fat-soluble vitamins A, D, E, and K. Similarly, organic, free-range eggs contain a third less cholesterol, a quarter less saturated fat, two times more omega-3 fatty acids, and three times more vitamin E than typical factory-farm eggs. As a bonus, these hormone-free and pastured meats are far leaner than those that come from penned and grain-fed animals, so we can enjoy red meat three times a week on our plan without guilt. These meats, especially the lamb and beef, tend to have a much more succulent flavor as well.

When it comes to fish, we prefer the smaller varieties such as wild salmon and tilapia because, in general, the bigger the fish, the greater the risk of toxicity. Plus, these fish are loaded with nutrients including selenium, magnesium, and B vitamins, along with inflammation-fighting and heart-healthy omega-3 fatty acids. A tiny can of sardines, for example, makes a terrific, low-calorie snack and contains a whopping two thousand milligrams of omega-3s, along with twenty-six grams of protein! We enjoy fish four times a week on our plan, but you can feel free to eat it more often; many of our clients who enjoy a six-ounce can of wild salmon as a snack every day find that the oils and collagen do wonders for their skin.

While vegetables and legumes do contain some of the essential amino acids, unlike animal protein, they do not contain them all. Therefore, while we do use lentils, chickpeas, and beans as a source of protein in several of our recipes, we believe that animal protein gives you the bigger nutritional hit. Beans and legumes can also cause bloating, so we limit them to one or two times a week.

If you are a vegetarian, there are a number of recipes in our plan that allow you to substitute organic tofu or tempeh for the chicken, turkey, or beef. When cooking with tofu, you should always opt for organic, *firm*—as opposed to silken—tofu, as the silken is highly processed and harder for your body to digest. With tempeh, you want to choose an organic variety that comes pre-marinated; we like Turtle Island Foods brand, and their sesame garlic and lemon pepper flavors work well in all our dishes.

Greens

As many servings as possible, especially of the powerhouse greens.

1 serving = 1 cup.

Dark green, leafy vegetables are, calorie for calorie, the most concentrated source of nutrition of any food. They deliver mega-doses of health-boosting vitamins (including K, C, E, and many of the B vitamins), minerals (including calcium, potassium, and magnesium), and phytonutrients (including beta-carotene and lutein, which protect our cells from damage and have anti-aging properties). The real standout among these is vitamin K, which helps to regulate blood sugar and protects against inflammation—and a single cup of most cooked greens provides at least *nine* times the minimum recommended daily intake. But the benefits of greens don't stop there: One cup of cooked kale, for example, not only provides 100 percent of your recommended daily allowance for vitamins K, A, and C, but also has antioxidant, anti-inflammatory, and natural detoxification benefits. In fact, new research shows that eating kale on a regular basis actually lowers your risk of five different types of cancer, including breast cancer. Greens are also low in carbs and high in fiber, which means they take longer to digest and won't spike your blood sugar—you'll stay full longer after eating them, and won't experience the sugar-crashes that lead to cravings.

The greens that we call the powerhouse greens are kale, spinach, collards, chard, and cabbage. All of these have amazingly potent nutritional, antioxidant, and anti-inflammatory benefits. Other healthy greens include dandelion, baby field greens, arugula, romaine lettuce, and watercress. We eat greens at least twice a day on our meal plan and sometimes more. In general, the powerhouse greens taste better when cooked, so we enjoy them steamed or sautéed with a variety of toppings; but we also enjoy a salad of raw greens at least once day. If you've never been a fan of greens, we've given you a number of tasty options that you won't be able to resist, such as Pumpkin-Raisin Collard Greens (page 256) or even our Simple Steamed Greens (page 258), which can be made with a variety of different seasonings. You'll be amazed at how a dash of toasted sesame oil or fresh ginger can liven up greens and make them melt in your mouth.

Other Vegetables

Two servings a day, or as many as you can eat.

1 serving = 1 cup.

Many vegetables run a close second to greens in terms of their nutritional value. You'll find the best ones in our meal plan: carrots, zucchini, sweet potatoes, onions, bell peppers, tomatoes, celery, scallions, cauliflower, parsnips, daikon radish, and mushrooms. Many of these vegetables contain important phytonutrients called carotenoids and flavonoids. These are the pigments that give them their bright and appealing colors, from the yellow found in a yellow bell pepper to the red in a tomato, and they have powerful antioxidant and anti-inflammatory properties. The more colorful your vegetables, the healthier you will be, and the less inflammation you will have throughout your body. Daikon radish, often featured in Asian cuisine, also aids in the digestion and metabolism of fats, so you can slice it into salads or try our Daikon Radish Relish (page 268) to give your fat-burning powers an extra boost. For the sweet vegetables—such as carrots and sweet potatoes—we recommend that you limit yourself to one serving a day, as they contain more sugar.

We also like sea vegetables such as kelp, nori, wakame, and kombu seaweeds, which are staples of the Asian diet and high in nutrients, including vitamins A, C, and E, and minerals such as calcium, magnesium, and potassium. They are also high in trace minerals—minerals that your body needs for optimum health, but in much smaller amounts, such as copper, iron, iodine, and zinc. We include the option to enjoy them as snacks, or to sprinkle them over certain of our dishes for an additional nutritional punch.

Fruits

One to two servings per day.

1 serving = 1 cup.

Fruits are an ideal source of healthy carbohydrates: They give you plenty of energy while still being relatively low in calories, and they are packed with vitamins, minerals, and fiber. Like vegetables, they also contain inflammation-fighting carotenoids and flavonoids, especially fruits that are deep reds, purples, and blues. In our plan, we like apples, pears, bananas, peaches, and any berries, especially blueberries. They are all great for satisfying your sweet tooth, so we often incorporate them into breakfasts and desserts, when many of us seek something sweet. Leaving the skin on any organic fruits will also give you an extra dose of healthy fiber. We also use black cherry concentrate in some of our marinades for meat—it's an easy and delicious way to add flavor to a dish and give your food an extra nutritional boost.

Grains

One to two servings a day.

1 serving = ½ cup.

Healthy grains are another good source of carbohydrates. Contrary to what some diets and weight-loss plans will tell you, carbs themselves are not responsible for weight gain. In fact, your body *needs* carbohydrates for energy, brain power, and a host of other functions. The problem is that most of us eat too many of the wrong kinds of carbs—namely, processed and refined grains such as wheat and corn that have been stripped of all fiber and nutritional value. Without a cushion of fiber and nutrients to slow the digestive process and help regulate blood sugar, these processed grains can be extremely taxing to the body, causing cravings, blood sugar spikes, and inflammation.

In our plan, we eat only small amounts of whole, unprocessed grains such as brown rice, oats, and quinoa that provide your body with an ample source of carbohydrates along with additional vitamins and fiber. Often referred to as a "supergrain," quinoa is not technically a grain at all, but a seed from a South American plant. It has a fluffy, slightly crunchy consistency when cooked and a delicious nutty flavor that makes it a perfect addition to any meal. It is also high in protein and, unlike most plants, contains all of the essential amino acids, along with a host of other health-building nutrients and antioxidants.

Dairy

No more than one serving a day.
1 serving = 1 tablespoon to ¼ cup.

Because cow's milk is both allergenic and high in calories, most dairy is off limits in our program. However, we love organic, grass-fed butter (also known as pasture butter) because it contains high levels of omega-3 fatty acids and a host of other vitamins, as well as antioxidant and immunity-boosting agents. Adding a little grass-fed butter to your cooking is an easy way to add both flavor and healthy fats without upping your calorie count—a teaspoon is only forty calories. Furthermore, your body needs saturated fat to absorb and process the fat-soluble vitamins D, E, and K, found in vegetables and greens, and to manufacture vitamin A. So adding a pat of butter to your steamed carrots or kale will ensure that you are getting as many nutrients from your veggies as possible.

We also enjoy small amounts of organic, whole-milk, full-fat Greek yogurt, which is minimally processed and easier for your body to digest than regular dairy because of its fermentation process. If you've never tried Greek yogurt, it is thicker and creamier than standard American yogurt and boasts an amazing array of health benefits. Not only is it loaded with calcium, B vitamins, potassium, and anti-inflammatory probiotics, but one serving also contains an impressive twenty grams of protein (regular yogurt contains ten to twelve grams) along with less than half the carbs and sugar.

We use unsweetened almond milk as a substitute for dairy in many of our breakfasts and smoothies. Far more nutritious than rice milk or soy milk, it provides 30 percent of your recommended daily value for calcium and 25 percent of your vitamin D. Plus, one cup has only sixty calories!

Healthy Fats

Four to five servings a day.

1 serving = 1 to 2 tablespoons.

In addition to helping you absorb key vitamins, healthy fats are an important energy source, especially when you're exercising regularly. In addition to organic, grass-fed butter, the other healthy fats we use throughout our meal plan include extra-virgin olive oil, toasted sesame oil, avocado, coconut, and various kinds of nuts, especially raw almonds, cashews, walnuts, and pecans.

Nuts in particular are a great, heart-healthy source of protein, omega-3 fatty acids, unsaturated fats, and fiber, so we use them frequently as snacks and toppings. We also like organic almond butter, which makes a fantastic dip or spread, as well as our own version of nut butter, Cashew Cream (page 267), which can be used as a healthy substitute for mayonnaise. You should always buy your nuts raw and unsalted. Seasoned nuts tend to be high in sodium, while you can never be sure what kinds of oils roasted nuts have been cooked in—and they tend to go rancid much more quickly. For those who prefer roasted nuts, we've given you a quick-and-easy recipe for Toasted Almonds (page 270) that delivers all the flavor of roasted almonds without the oil. Toasted Coconut (page 271) adds a touch of sweetness to several of our desserts.

Seeds are another excellent source of healthy fats, omega-3s, and many other nutrients, including iron and folic acid. Our Toasted Pumpkin Seeds (page 271) make a terrific topping for salads and cooked greens, as do raw sesame seeds, which actually contain more calcium than milk!

Herbs and Seasonings

As many as you like.

Fresh or dried organic herbs are an easy way to add more nutrients and flavor to any dish while adding very few calories. We use them liberally throughout our meal plan, and you can feel free to add even more if you'd like. Parsley, dill, oregano, basil, thyme, cilantro, rosemary, sage, and mint all feature prominently, as do plenty of other seasonings such as garlic, ginger, red pepper, cayenne pepper, turmeric, curry, and sea salt.

Many of these herbs and seasonings have powerful antioxidant and anti-inflammatory properties that will help you shed false fat and boost your overall health, as does sea salt, which contains natural iodine as well as fifty trace minerals not found in processed table salt. We also use sweeter spices, such as cinnamon and cloves, which can provide a healthy fix for sugar cravings. Just sprinkle them over a piece of fruit or a bowl of quinoa for a simple snack that will satisfy your sweet tooth.

Sweeteners

Sparingly.

1 serving = 1 teaspoon, or 1 tablespoon at most.

In place of sugars and artificial sweeteners (even aspartame-free Splenda and the "natural" sweetener Truvia are highly processed and contain chemicals that are toxic to the body), we use raw honey and grade B maple syrup because they are found in nature and are minimally processed. We also use organic vanilla extract in some of our breakfasts and desserts. Organic vanillas are not only free from the additional sugar and chemicals found in commercial vanillas, but they also give desserts a much richer flavor. Yum!

Step 3: Choose Organic and Local Foods Whenever Possible

Much has been said in recent years about the enormous health benefits of eating organic. Organic foods are farmed without the use of synthetic pesticides, chemical fertilizers, or genetically engineered ingredients, and once harvested they are minimally processed without artificial ingredients, preservatives, or irradiation. We're aiming to eliminate toxins from your diet and focus on high-quality, macronutrient-rich foods—and buying organic produce, grains, and meats whenever you can will greatly facilitate this process. These days, organic products are widely available at specialty markets like Whole Foods or Trader Joe's, at health food stores, and at most chain supermarkets as well, often at lower prices. If you are having trouble finding a particular organic product, your next best option is to look for one that is clearly labeled NO ARTIFICIAL INGREDIENTS or NO GMOS (genetically modified organisms). With meats, you should always opt for cuts that are hormone- and antibiotic-free, free-range, or grass-fed.

When it comes to the recipes in this book, you should assume that all fresh fruits and vegetables are organic, all meats and eggs are organic (or at least no-hormone, no-antibiotic, and free-range), and that any other ingredients—such as chicken broth, tamari, and spices—are organic as well, even if it isn't specified on the ingredients list. If you are unable to find the organic version of a particular ingredient, don't worry—just choose the most natural, unprocessed option available.

In addition, locally grown produce will have a much higher nutrient value because it is harvested at the peak of ripeness (as opposed to foods that are shipped over long distances, which are harvested several weeks prior). You can find a variety of locally grown foods at your neighborhood Whole Foods or farmer's market. Buying local and organic is the very best you can do for your body, so for these two weeks at least, we recommend that you give it a try.

Step 4: Prepare Your Foods the Right Way

When it comes to cooking vegetables—both greens and others—we strongly recommend steaming over boiling, as it leads to better nutrient retention. Steaming also seals in the flavor of your vegetables, and eliminates the need for fats and oils during preparation. To steam your veggies, simply place your food in a covered, perforated steamer basket that rests above a pot of boiling water. Our recipe for Simple Steamed Greens on page 258 provides you with directions and cook times for a variety of greens. When it comes to other vegetables, you want to be sure not to steam them too long—they should be slightly tender but not mushy.

Stir-frying, sautéing, baking, and broiling are other reasonably healthy ways to prepare meat and vegetables, as they require very little or no additional fats. With stir-frying, you cook your food on high heat for a very short amount of time, stirring frequently and using only a very small amount of oil. Sautéing is usually done over medium heat and traditionally requires more butter or oil to prevent sticking, but our recipes work around this by using a splash of organic low-sodium chicken broth to extend the cook time rather than adding more fat. Broiling and baking both require no additional oil, although we do use healthy marinades to keep the food moist and add a burst of nutrients and flavor to the dishes. Broiling gets extra points because, like grilling, it allows excess fat to drip away from the food. Just be careful not to char your meats by broiling them for too long—blackened or burned food is toxic, so watch your meats closely and remove them from the oven when they are seared but not charred.

When cooking on the stovetop with fats and oils, you always want to avoid heating them to the smoking point, since this can cause them to break down into unhealthy components. We want to preserve all the healthy omega-3 fatty acids in the olive oil and butter we use for cooking.

Step 5: Drink Water, Water, Water!

You should drink half your weight in ounces of water a day, especially when you're exercising regularly. This means that if you weigh 140 pounds, you want to aim for roughly seventy ounces, or eight to nine standard eight-ounce glasses. The most important water is the "morning water"—a one- to two-glass serving of room-temperature water that you drink the moment you wake up to provide a soothing cleanse for your system and to flush out any toxins. You can add a splash of fresh lemon or lime juice if you like—citrus is a natural detoxifier.

We recommend that while on the program, you keep a bottle of water with you throughout the day to remind yourself to stay hydrated. If plain water is uninspiring and you're having trouble consuming your requisite amount of H_2O, try one of the coolers on page 272 in the beverage section of our recipes. Better than any store-bought, flavored waters, our all-natural coolers are wonderfully refreshing and provide a dose of vitamins and antioxidants as well. They are also a great substitute for snacking if you ever have a sugar craving—they will fill you up and clear your head far more effectively than that afternoon candy bar.

The Physique 57 Kitchen Makeover

Before you start our two-week program, we recommend that you take stock of your kitchen and get rid of the old to make room for the new: new ingredients, new ways of eating, and new and healthier ways of preparing food. Here are five easy ways to conduct your very own Kitchen Makeover:

1. **Jettison the junk.** Start by going through your pantry and kitchen cabinets to get rid of any food that is not a part of your new lifestyle. This means any processed and packaged foods that contain high levels of sugars, unhealthy fats, or artificial ingredients, which you are now trying to avoid. Don't forget any secret stashes of junk food such as candies in your desk drawer at work. Here are some of the items you'll want to be sure to toss:

   - Any diet-based foods that are labeled DIET, LOW-FAT, or SUGAR-FREE
   - Any artificial sweeteners such as Splenda
   - Sodas, bottled iced teas and coffees, and any other unhealthy, sugary beverages
   - Store-bought, non-organic condiments like ketchup and mayonnaise
   - Store-bought salad dressings—most of these, even the "healthy" brands, actually have a ton of sugar
   - Anything with wheat or processed grains
   - Milk, ice cream, and other forms of highly processed, non-organic dairy
   - Fake, nonfermented soy—many of today's popular soy foods such as soy dogs or soy chips are so heavily processed, they barely resemble food
   - Poor quality, non-organic oils including corn and vegetable oils
   - Cooking sprays—these contain propellant, a chemical component used in lighter fluid that has no place in the body
   - Any fake foods with artificial colors

2. **Check your equipment.** Cooking is made far easier by having the proper tools. To prepare the recipes in this book, you'll need: a food processor or blender, one proper chef's knife, a wooden or bamboo cutting board, a baking sheet, a medium skillet, a large skillet with a lid, a few sauce pots,

a steamer basket, a mesh strainer, a glass pitcher, and a set of mixing bowls: small, medium, and large. When it comes to pots and pans, we prefer stainless steel. Stainless steel has no chemicals, so you don't need to worry about scratching the Teflon as with nonstick pans; it's also lighter than copper, cast iron, or ceramic. Plus, the cleanup is very easy with stainless—you can just throw dishes in the dishwasher. We also like glass jars or small Pyrex bowls for storage.

3. **Get organized.** You'll want to clear the counters as much as possible to give yourself plenty of space, and possibly rearrange your cupboards to have some foods close at hand so you can reach for them when cooking. We like to have sea salt, pepper, and other spices and seasonings within reach of the stove. However, your delicate oils should be kept away from heat—if possible, in the fridge.

4. **Throw out the microwave**—or at least put a pretty dish towel over it! Microwaves heat food by exploding the water molecules, so you are changing the food on a molecular level. For these two weeks, we urge you to avoid the microwave if possible—reheat on the stovetop or in the oven when you can.

5. **Stock up.** Now that you've removed all the foods that don't serve your purpose over the next two weeks, you're ready to stock up on those that do. The box on page 211 provides a list of the staples and nonperishable items that you'll want on your shelves; depending on how often you cook, you may already have quite a few of them. Before you begin the program, we recommend that you review this list and make note of any items you will need to purchase along with the perishable and more specific items (like meat and produce) that you will buy for the recipes each week. Remember to upgrade your pantry staples and buy organic whenever possible!

And now it's time to take a look at the mouthwatering meals you will enjoy as you transform your body in the weeks ahead. As you'll see from the daily menus laid out in chapter 13, eating healthy—and nourishing your body in the best possible way—has never been so much fun!

In Your Pantry

Before going to the store for the first time, check your shelves to be sure you have the following basic ingredients. Again, we recommend that you buy organic whenever possible.

Condiments:

Grass-fed or pasture butter (we like Kate's brand best)

Extra-virgin olive oil

Toasted sesame oil

Balsamic vinegar

Brown rice vinegar

Cider vinegar

Brown mustard

Dijon mustard

Olive oil mayonnaise (we like Spectrum brand)

Hot sauce (we like Melinda's brand)

Mild salsa (we like Muir Glen brand)

Mirin (sweet rice wine)

Tamari

Unsweetened almond butter

Peach preserves (100 percent fruit with no added sugar)

Grade B maple syrup

Raw honey

Black cherry concentrate (we like Dynamic Health brand)

Dried Herbs and Spices:

Basil

Cardamom

Cayenne pepper

Celery seeds

(continued)

✓Chili powder

✓ Cinnamon

✓Cloves

 Coriander

 Cumin

 Curry powder

 Dill

✓ Fennel

✓Freshly ground black pepper

✓ Garlic powder

 Ground fennel

✓Ground ginger

✓ Italian seasoning

 Marjoram

 Minced onion

 No-salt, all-purpose seasoning (we like Simply Organic brand)

✓Nutmeg

✓Onion powder

 Oregano

✓Paprika

 Poultry seasoning

✓Red pepper flakes

✓Rosemary

 Sage

✓Sea salt (we like Celtic or Redmond Real brand)

 Thyme

✓Turmeric

Grains:

 Brown rice

 Quinoa

Rolled oats

Gluten-free crackers

Nuts:

Chopped walnuts

Chopped pecans

Raw cashews

Raw, sliced almonds

Miscellaneous:

Raisins

Raw pumpkin seeds (also called *pepitas*)

Unsweetened applesauce

Unsweetened cocoa powder

Unsweetened shredded coconut

Pumpkin, canned (*not* pumpkin pie filling)

Vanilla extract

Green tea

Instant herbal or grain "coffee" (we like Teeccino, Cafix, or Roma brands; Teeccino and Roma are caffeine-free)

Low-sodium chicken broth

Low-sodium vegetable broth

Anchovies, jarred or canned

Roasted sweet peppers, jarred

Wild salmon, canned

Light coconut milk

Sweet white miso paste

Nori strips (we like Annie Chun's brand)

Wakame seaweed

12

WHAT'S COOKING?

THE DAILY MEAL PLANS WE HAVE CREATED FOR THIS book are designed to give you plenty of delicious food to keep you going throughout the day. We enjoy four different meals: breakfast, lunch, an afternoon snack, and dinner accompanied by dessert. You'll be eating two servings of healthy high-fiber grains, three servings of lean protein, and at least seven servings of fruit and vegetables a day. If that sounds like a lot of food, it is! But our goal is to satisfy both your stomach and your taste buds so that you never feel deprived.

As you read through the meal plans and recipes, you will likely find that there are some dishes that appeal to you more than others. If so, feel free to swap out one lunch for a different lunch, or one dinner for another—each is as good as the next. The only thing we recommend is that you NOT have red meat more than three times a week; while we encourage you to enjoy lean, grass-fed lamb and beef, eating it too often will give you more cholesterol and saturated fat than your body needs. So if you can, try to swap poultry for poultry, or fish for fish—you'll stay closer to your ideal caloric intake and ensure that you're getting all the essential vitamins and nutrients in the proper portions. You can also feel free to swap around any of the snacks and substitute ones from the list below.

For each week, we've also provided a list of sides, condiments, and toppings that can be made in advance to help you save time. These easy-to-make foods, such as Caramelized Onions and Cashew Cream, appear in many of the recipes and can also be used to spice up other snacks and dishes as you see fit. And for those of you who barely have time to sleep, let alone cook (we both fall into this category from time to time), the Girl-on-the-Go section on page 221 provides a list of healthy choices for eating out, and shows you how easy it can be to eat the Physique 57 way wherever you are. You can use these suggestions anytime you're in a pinch during the initial two-week program, as well as after the first two weeks to help you maintain your newly gorgeous physique.

ENERGY BOOSTERS: HEALTHY SNACKS TO KEEP YOU GOING

Anytime you feel hungry or need a pick-me-up, especially prior to your workouts, you can reach for any of the healthy snacks listed below. While these foods do contain calories, they are also packed with nutrients and fiber to help you fill up quickly. Our meal plan provides a suggested snack for each day, but you can feel free to substitute any other snack from this list that you prefer.

- 1 handful raw almonds (about 15 nuts) with 1 tablespoon raisins.
- ½ cup unsweetened applesauce sprinkled with cinnamon and either 1 tablespoon Toasted Almonds (page 270) or 1 tablespoon raisins.
- Apple slices (skin on) dipped in raw honey and Toasted Pumpkin Seeds (page 271).
- Apple slices (skin on) with either 1 tablespoon almond butter, 2 tablespoons Cashew Cream (page 267), or 2 tablespoons Cocoa Cream (page 267).
- ½ avocado, drizzled with 1 teaspoon olive oil, pinch sea salt, and ground black pepper.
- ½ banana with 2 tablespoons Cocoa Cream (page 267).
- Celery sticks with 1 tablespoon almond butter and 1 tablespoon raisins.
- Chai Latte (page 272).
- Crudités—such as broccoli florets, carrot sticks, celery sticks, cherry tomatoes, or bell pepper strips—dipped in 2 tablespoons Cashew Cream (page 267).

(continued)

- Crudités with 2 tablespoons store-bought organic hummus.
- Crudités with 2 tablespoons Lemon Ginger Tahini Sauce (page 269).
- Crudités with 2 tablespoons Onion Dip (page 270).
- Deviled egg: Remove yolk and mash to combine with 1 teaspoon Caramelized Onions (page 266). Place "deviled" yolk back in egg and top with freshly ground black pepper.
- Frozen grapes (15) and raw almonds (12).
- Green juices. For an extra serving of powerhouse greens, try a green juice from your local health food store or juice bar. Kale, collards, and dandelion all work well, and you can add a small amount of beet, carrot, or green apple to make it sweet. Because raw, uncooked, dark greens are more difficult to digest than cooked ones, we recommend limiting green juices to once or twice a week.
- Green tea.
- Hard-boiled egg with sea salt.
- Hot Chocolate (page 273).
- Kale Chips (page 255, or try Ed's of Maine, available at health food stores).
- Latte (page 273).
- 5 to 10 all-natural, gluten-free or brown rice crackers (Mary's Gone Crackers brand is our favorite) with either 1 tablespoon almond butter, 2 tablespoons Cashew Cream (page 267), or 2 tablespoons Onion Dip (page 270).
- Pear slices (skin on) with either 1 tablespoon almond butter, 2 tablespoons Cashew Cream (page 267), or 2 tablespoons Cocoa Cream (page 267).
- Nori strips (we like Annie Chun's brand, especially the wasabi or toasted sesame flavor).
- 1 (6-ounce) can smoked, skinless, boneless sardines packed in olive oil (we like Bela or Crown Prince brand), either plain or over 5 to 10 gluten-free crackers.
- Smoothie (page 274).
- Sorbet popsicles (left over from desserts, page 262).
- 1 can (6 ounces) wild salmon mixed with 1 tablespoon olive oil mayonnaise.

WEEK ONE

TIME-SAVERS: FOODS TO PREPARE AHEAD

- Basic Quinoa (page 253)
- Caramelized Onions (page 266)
- Cashew Cream (page 267)
- Garlicky Lime Dressing (page 268)
- Kale Chips (page 255)
- Miso-Sesame Dressing (page 269)
- Onion Dip (page 270)
- Toasted Almonds (page 270)
- Toasted Pumpkin Seeds (page 271)

Day 1
Breakfast: Basic Oats, Chai Tea Latte
Lunch: Mediterranean Turkey Lettuce Wrap, ½ cup Basic Quinoa, Kale Chips
Snack: Apple with 2 tablespoons almond butter
Dinner: Baked Tilapia with Daikon Radish Relish, Simple Steamed Spinach, Baked Sweet Potato
Dessert: Banana Smoothie

Day 2
Breakfast: Hard-Boiled Eggs Florentine, Latte
Lunch: Turkey Burgers, Miso-Sesame Salad
Snack: 5 to 10 gluten-free crackers with Cashew Cream
Dinner: BBQ Chicken, ½ cup brown rice, Simple Steamed Collard Greens
Dessert: Crustless Cherry Pie

Day 3
Breakfast: Yogurt Berry Parfait, green tea
Lunch: "Taco" Salad
Snack: 1 can (6 ounces) wild salmon with 1 tablespoon olive oil mayonnaise
Dinner: Ginger Shrimp & Cabbage Stir-Fry, ½ cup brown rice
Dessert: Vanilla-Scented Poached Pears

Day 4
Breakfast: Personal Frittatas, Latte
Lunch: Southwest Bean Salad
Snack: Carrot sticks with Onion Dip
Dinner: Roast Turkey Breast, Pumpkin-Quinoa Risotto, Simple Steamed Kale
Dessert: Cocoa-Dipped Banana with Toasted Coconut

Day 5
Breakfast: Carrot Grain Omelet, Hot Chocolate
Lunch: Steak Salad with Tomatoes & Avocado
Snack: ½ cup unsweetened applesauce with 1 tablespoon Toasted Almonds and cinnamon
Dinner: Cuban Chicken
Dessert: Blueberry Sorbet

Day 6
Breakfast: Spinach Scramble, Latte
Lunch: Chicken Salad
Snack: 5 to 10 gluten-free crackers with 1 tablespoon almond butter
Dinner: Aromatic Lamb with Vegetables, ½ cup brown rice
Dessert: Chilled Honeydew Soup

Day 7
Breakfast: Vanilla Oatmeal with Raisins, Chai Latte
Lunch: Wild Salmon Salad
Snack: Sliced bell peppers with Onion Dip
Dinner: Herbed Maple Chicken, ½ cup quinoa, Pumpkin-Raisin Collard Greens
Dessert: Chocolate-Covered Strawberries

WEEK TWO

TIME SAVERS: FOODS TO PREPARE AHEAD

- Basic Quinoa (page 253)
- Caramelized Onions (page 266)
- Cashew Cream (page 267)
- Garlicky Lime Dressing (page 268)
- Honey Mustard Dressing (page 268)
- Kale Chips (page 255)
- Onion Dip (page 270)
- Toasted Almonds (page 270)
- Toasted Pumpkin Seeds (page 271)

Day 8

Breakfast: Breakfast Egg Salad, green tea

Lunch: Turkey Eggplant Napoleon, Spinach Salad with Honey Mustard Dressing

Snack: Apple with honey and Toasted Pumpkin Seeds

Dinner: Lemon Snapper with Daikon Radish Relish, Simple Steamed Spinach, ½ cup quinoa

Dessert: Baked Bananas with Vanilla-Maple Syrup

Day 9

Breakfast: Basic Oats, Hot Chocolate

Lunch: Caesar Salad

Snack: 1 can (6 ounces) wild salmon with 1 tablespoon olive oil mayonnaise

Dinner: Grilled Grass-Fed London Broil, Roasted Cauliflower, Simple Steamed Swiss Chard

Dessert: Raspberry Melon Parfait

Day 10

Breakfast: Green Pancakes, Latte

Lunch: Pear-Arugula Salad with Chicken & Walnuts

Snack: 5 to 10 gluten-free crackers with Cashew Cream

Dinner: Citrus Shrimp over Garlicky Lime Salad (with baby spinach), Baked Sweet Potato

Dessert: Baked Apples

Day 11
Breakfast: Maple-Cinnamon Porridge, Hot Chocolate
Lunch: Green Lentils with Shiitake Mushrooms
Snack: Nori strips
Dinner: Beef & Quinoa Stuffed Peppers
Dessert: Peach Sorbet

Day 12
Breakfast: Sausage & Veggie Plate, green tea
Lunch: Easy "Tortilla" Soup, Garlicky Lime Salad
Snack: Celery sticks with 1 tablespoon almond butter and 1 tablespoon raisins
Dinner: Herbed Salmon with Daikon Radish Relish, Basic Quinoa, Simple Steamed Kale
Dessert: Cocoa-Dipped Banana with Toasted Coconut

Day 13
Breakfast: Yogurt Berry Parfait, Chai Latte
Lunch: Quinoa Pilaf
Snack: Kale Chips
Dinner: Braised Chicken with Black Cherry Shallot Sauce, Roasted Butternut Squash, Simple Steamed Swiss Chard
Dessert: Orange Sherbet

Day 14
Breakfast: Breakfast Egg Salad, Latte
Lunch: Chicken Lettuce Wrap, Tomato-Cucumber Salad
Snack: 5 to 10 gluten-free crackers with Onion Dip
Dinner: Turkey Curry served over Basic Quinoa, Simple Steamed Spinach
Dessert: Watermelon Refresher

GIRL ON THE GO: TIPS FOR EATING OUT WHEN YOU CAN'T COOK IN

No matter how hard you try, there will always be days when preparing three meals from scratch just isn't feasible. But if you are proactive and resourceful, you'll find that it's fairly easy to follow the Physique 57 rules for healthy eating wherever you are. Many of the dishes on our meal plan can be re-created using the standard offerings at any restaurant or take-out venue. Just keep our eating guidelines in mind when you order: Avoid unhealthy processed and allergenic foods, steer clear of the calorie culprits on pages 197 and 198, and skip most grains and dairy, loading up instead on lean protein, greens, vegetables, and fruits.

To help you approximate the meal plan as closely as possible when dining out or grabbing food on the go, we've created a simple formula for every meal that you can use to help you choose the right foods in the proper portions. We've also come up with a list of healthy options for breakfasts, lunches, dinners, and desserts—all Physique 57 friendly, and no cooking required!

Breakfast = 1 serving whole grains OR dairy + 1 serving fruit + 1 serving lean protein

- Instant organic rolled oats (buy the packets and make them with hot water from Starbucks or your office coffee machine), with 1 banana or 1 cup fruit and 1 handful raw almonds.
- Spinach omelet with fruit on the side.
- 2 hard-boiled eggs with 1 banana or 1 cup other fruit.
- 1 cup fruit with ¼ cup whole-milk Greek yogurt and 1 handful almonds.

Girl-on-the-Go Tips

- *When eating out, watch your portions: Most restaurants will give you three or four eggs in an omelet and two cups of cooked oatmeal, so eat half of whatever they serve.*
- *Stay clear of refined grains and carbohydrates: No toast, muffins, bagels, or the like.*

(continued)

Lunch = 3 servings greens + 1 serving lean protein + 1 additional serving vegetables

■ A big salad with either grilled chicken or fish, 4 slices deli turkey, 1 can (6 ounces) wild salmon, or 1 hard-boiled egg on top and lots of veggies (you can always ask the chef to hold any unhealthy ingredients like cheese, bacon, or croutons).

■ Turkey or veggie burger on a bed of greens or with a side salad.

■ Hummus and vegetable plate with side salad.

■ A vegetable, broth-based soup (never cream) with grilled chicken or fish and a side salad.

■ Taco salad with lettuce, salsa, and grilled chicken, fish, or black beans—just order it without the taco shell, sour cream, and cheese.

Girl-on-the-Go Tip

• *Always ask for your salad dressing on the side and then dip your greens and veggies—you'll use far less dressing this way. Better yet, make your own dressing using 1 tablespoon olive oil, 2 tablespoons vinegar, a squeeze of fresh lemon, and a little sea salt.*

Dinner = 1 serving lean protein + 1 serving greens + 2 servings vegetables

■ Grilled chicken, fish, or shrimp with brown rice and steamed vegetables on the side (you can get this at any Chinese restaurant). Dress this up with a squeeze of lemon or your own organic tamari.

■ Chicken paillard: grilled chicken breast with arugula and tomatoes on top—a staple at French restaurants.

■ Grilled chicken fajitas with black beans, vegetables, and fresh salsa with a side salad. You can ask the chef to hold the tortillas, sour cream, and other toppings.

■ Sushi or sashimi with brown rice, steamed vegetables, and a seaweed salad, dressing on the side. You can use your own organic tamari.

Girl-on-the-Go Tips

- *Instead of an appetizer, order an extra serving of greens or veggies.*
- *If a dish comes with a sauce, ask for it on the side or skip it altogether—the base of most restaurant sauces is butter or hidden oil. Instead, ask the chef to prepare your dish with lemon or lime and salt and pepper.*
- *If a dish comes with a carb or pasta, ask for steamed vegetables instead.*
- *Avoid fried foods at all costs: Stick with steamed and grilled instead.*

Dessert = 1 serving fruit

■ Berries or fruit plate.

Girl-on-the-Go Tips

- *Although we enjoy sorbets on our meal plan, you should avoid the ones you find in restaurants—while low-fat and dairy-free, they are usually high in sugar.*
- *If your restaurant does not offer fruit, sip a green or herbal tea instead.*

13

KITCHEN DIVA

AT PHYSIQUE 57, WE BELIEVE THAT FOOD SHOULD BE about more than just losing weight, so we feel strongly that the process of preparing and eating your food should be something you enjoy. The recipes in this chapter are designed to open up a whole new world of culinary delights and show you just how easy it is to make tasty, healthy meals in your own kitchen every day. Even if you normally subsist on takeout, or skip meals altogether because you're in a rush, this chapter will transform you into a veritable Kitchen Diva, whipping up your own delicious dishes and savoring every bite!

The recipes in this chapter are incredibly simple and easy to adapt to your or your family's needs. Our breakfast and lunch recipes serve one, and all of the dinners and desserts serve two. If you're dining solo, you can simply cut the dinner recipes in half, or make the full recipe and save one portion for later in the week. All of the dinners are interchangeable, as are the lunches, so you can feel free to swap one recipe for another depending on your tastes. And all of the recipes are easily doubled, so you can use them for entertaining, or make and freeze extra portions for those days and evenings when you're in a rush.

The vegetarian recipes and those with a vegetarian option are highlighted with a V symbol next to the name. You can also modify any of the recipes on your own to make them vegetarian—for example, you can substitute a vegetable stock or broth anytime a recipe calls for chicken broth. As long as the amounts remain the same, you will not increase the calorie count.

So now it's time to roll up your sleeves, head to the kitchen, and start cooking! We hope that you enjoy these recipes, and that they will continue to grace your table for many years to come.

KITCHEN TIME SAVERS

As you are preparing the recipes, there are a number of easy substitutions you can make to save time and eliminate steps. All of these items can be found at your local supermarket or health food markets.

- For brown rice or quinoa: Instead of making rice or quinoa from scratch, use the frozen brown rice packets from Trader Joe's, Gogo organic rice bowls, or any other kind of instant, organic brown rice.
- For cooked chicken: Substitute an organic or no-hormone, no-antibiotic rotisserie chicken for cooked chicken or turkey in our salad and lunch recipes.
- For cooked turkey: You can substitute four or five thin slices of no-hormone, no-antibiotic, all-natural deli turkey for our salad and lunch recipes. We like Applegate Farms.
- For greens: Buy bagged, pre-washed organic greens for your salads whenever you can. Baby spinach also works for steaming. You can wash and prep your dinner greens ahead of time, even a few days in advance—just remove the stems, wash the leaves, and place them in a ziplock bag with a damp paper towel to preserve moisture.

BREAKFASTS

BASIC OATS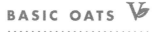

MAKES 1 SERVING

Basic Oats make the perfect, easy breakfast and can be enjoyed with a variety of healthy, flavorful toppings.

¾ cup unsweetened almond milk

½ cup rolled oats

1 teaspoon butter

Pinch sea salt

Place all the ingredients in a small saucepan and bring to a near boil (steaming and bubbly, but *not* a roaring boil—that would damage the almond milk and make it separate). Remove from the heat, cover with a lid, and let stand for 5 minutes.

KITCHEN DIVA TIP

Spice up your oats with one or more of the following:

- 1 tablespoon raisins
- 1 teaspoon grade B maple syrup or raw honey
- 1 tablespoon raw nuts (your choice)
- A sprinkle of cinnamon, nutmeg, or cloves
- ¼ cup unsweetened applesauce
- ½ banana, sliced
- ½ cup berries
- 1 teaspoon fruit-only jam

BREAKFAST EGG SALAD

MAKES 1 SERVING

1 hard-boiled egg

¼ cup cooked quinoa (page 253)

½ cup steamed kale (page 258)

1 teaspoon olive oil

Sea salt and freshly ground black pepper to taste

Chop the hard-boiled egg. In a small bowl, combine the chopped egg, quinoa, kale, oil, and salt and pepper. Mix well.

CARROT GRAIN OMELET

MAKES 1 SERVING

1 teaspoon olive oil

¼–½ cup shredded carrots

¼ teaspoon onion powder

Pinch sea salt

Freshly ground black pepper to taste

2 eggs

¼ cup cooked quinoa (page 253)

1 teaspoon butter

Heat the oil in a medium sauté pan and add the carrots, onion powder, sea salt, and pepper. Cook until the carrots are soft, about 4 minutes. In a small bowl, whisk the eggs and then add the cooked carrots and quinoa. Mix well.

In the same sauté pan, melt the butter over medium heat. Pour in the egg mixture, turn the heat to low, cover the pan with a lid, and cook on low for about 2 minutes. Then turn the pancake over and continue to cook until it is firm and cooked through, about another minute or two on the lowest setting. Remove from the heat, fold in half, and serve.

KITCHEN DIVA TIP

To make a perfect hard-boiled egg, place the egg in a pot covered with 2 inches of water and bring to a boil. Once a full rolling boil is achieved, cover the pot, remove it from the stove, and let it stand for 12 minutes. Submerge the egg in cold water for 3 minutes. Once the egg has cooled, crack it on a hard surface, and then roll to easily release the shell.

GREEN PANCAKES
· ·

MAKES 1 SERVING

To give these delicious pancakes an extra nutritional punch, add ½ teaspoon spirulina (blue-green algae) powder, available at health food stores. Garnish with any brightly colored fruit for a particularly striking dish.

> 2 eggs, beaten
> ¾ cup steamed kale (page 258)
> ½ cup cooked quinoa (page 253)
> ½ teaspoon spirulina powder (optional)
> 1 teaspoon dried chives or dried minced onion
> Sea salt and freshly ground black pepper to taste
> 1 teaspoon butter

Combine all the ingredients except the butter in a food processor and blend until smooth. Melt the butter in a sauté pan over medium heat, then ladle the mixture into the pan to make pancakes of your desired size. Turn the heat to low and cook the pancakes, lifting the edges to check progress. When the pancakes start to brown, flip them over using a spatula and cook on the other side until set.

HARD-BOILED EGGS FLORENTINE
· ·

MAKES 1 SERVING

This recipe works best if the eggs are newly cooked and slightly warm. For directions on how to make a perfect hard-boiled egg, see our Kitchen Diva Tip on page 227.

> 2 hard-boiled eggs
> ½ cup steamed spinach (page 258)
> ¼ cup Caramelized Onions (page 266)
> Sea salt and freshly ground black pepper to taste

Slice the eggs in half lengthwise. Puree the spinach and onions in a food processor, then heat in a small sauce pot and spoon over the eggs. Season to taste.

MAPLE-CINNAMON PORRIDGE V⃗

MAKES 1 SERVING

¾ cup cooked quinoa (page 253) or cooked brown rice

½ cup unsweetened almond milk

2 teaspoons grade B maple syrup

1 teaspoon butter

¼ teaspoon cinnamon

Splash vanilla extract

Place all the ingredients in a small saucepan and bring to a near boil (steaming and bubbly, but *not* a roaring boil, which would damage the almond milk and make it separate). Simmer for 5 minutes and then remove from the heat.

PERSONAL FRITTATAS V⃗

MAKES 1 SERVING

This recipe is a great way to use up any leftover vegetables—simply substitute ⅓ cup cooked vegetables of your choice for the greens or bell pepper.

3 button mushrooms, sliced

⅓ cup cooked spinach or kale (page 258) *or* ⅓ cup chopped red bell pepper

1 teaspoon olive oil

¼ cup Caramelized Onions (page 266)

2 eggs

Dash no-salt, all-purpose seasoning

Sea salt and freshly ground black pepper to taste

Preheat the oven to 350°.

Lightly sauté the mushrooms and spinach/red bell pepper in olive oil over medium-high heat until soft, about 2 to 5 minutes, stirring frequently.

Place three paper cupcake holders in a muffin tin and fill with equal amounts of the

(continued)

sautéed vegetables and onions. In a small bowl, whisk the eggs and season with the dash of all-purpose seasoning, salt, and pepper. Pour the eggs evenly over each of the muffin cups, and bake for about 15 to 20 minutes until firm and golden brown.

SAUSAGE & VEGGIE PLATE

MAKES 1 SERVING

When it comes to sausages, we like Bilinski's and Applegate Farms brands best—not only are they organic and super-tasty, but they also contain an impressive eight to eleven grams of protein per link!

- 1 link turkey or chicken sausage, sliced into ¼" disks
- 1 teaspoon butter
- 1 cup of any chopped vegetable (kale, broccoli, spinach, carrots, and cauliflower are all good options)
- ¼ cup low-sodium chicken broth as needed

Sauté the sausage in butter on medium heat until it turns golden brown. Add the vegetables and continue to cook, adding broth as needed to keep the sausage and vegetables from sticking to the pan, until the vegetables are fully cooked, about 5 minutes.

SPINACH SCRAMBLE ⱽ

MAKES 1 SERVING

- 2 eggs
- 1 cup pre-washed baby spinach
- 1 teaspoon butter
- Sea salt and freshly ground black pepper to taste

Whisk the eggs together in a small bowl. In a medium pan, sauté the spinach in butter over medium heat until wilted. Add the eggs and scramble together until cooked. Add sea salt and pepper to taste.

VANILLA OATMEAL WITH RAISINS

MAKES 1 SERVING

½ cup rolled oats

1 cup filtered water

1 tablespoon full-fat Greek yogurt

2 tablespoons slivered raw almonds

1 teaspoon grade B maple syrup

1 teaspoon vanilla extract

1 tablespoon raisins or chopped dates

Sea salt to taste

Combine all ingredients and bring to a boil. Reduce the heat and simmer for about 1 to 2 minutes until the oatmeal thickens, stirring occasionally.

YOGURT BERRY PARFAIT

MAKES 1 SERVING

¾ cup cooked Basic Oats (page 226)

½ cup fresh blueberries *or* ½ cup chopped apple (skin on) *or* ½ banana, sliced

¼ cup full-fat Greek yogurt

1 tablespoon raw slivered almonds

1 teaspoon grade B maple syrup or raw honey

KITCHEN DIVA TIP

Instead of raw, slivered almonds, try the Toasted Almonds on page 270.

Layer one-half of the oats, one-half of the fruit, and one-half of the yogurt into a parfait glass or small bowl. Repeat one more time: oats, then fruit, then yogurt. Top with the almonds and drizzle with syrup or honey.

LUNCHES

CAESAR SALAD
....

MAKES 1 SERVING

This refreshing version of a Caesar salad is every bit as tasty as the original without the processed, unhealthy fats. For an extra dose of nutrients, sprinkle shredded nori or spirulina powder on top.

For the dressing:

¼ cup raw cashews

¼ cup water

1 clove garlic, crushed

1 tablespoon fresh lemon juice

1 tablespoon olive oil

Pinch sea salt

1 teaspoon granulated kelp (optional)

Freshly ground black pepper to taste

1 tablespoon anchovies

For the salad:

½ cup shredded cooked chicken (about 4 ounces)

3 cups shredded romaine lettuce

Mix all the dressing ingredients in a food processor. Toss with the chicken and romaine and serve.

CHICKEN LETTUCE WRAP

MAKES 1 SERVING

¾ cup cooked chicken, shredded (about 5 ounces)

2 tablespoons Cashew Cream (page 267)

2 tablespoons diced celery

Dash no-salt, all-purpose seasoning

3 large romaine lettuce leaves

¼ cup Caramelized Onions (page 266)

Sea salt and freshly ground black pepper to taste

VEGETARIAN OPTION

You can substitute ¾ cup chopped, store-bought marinated tempeh for the chicken. Prepare in the same way.

In a small bowl, combine the chicken, Cashew Cream, celery, and seasoning. Arrange the three lettuce leaves on a plate and place an equal amount of the chicken mixture and onions on each. Season with salt and pepper. Fold the lettuce around the mixture to form a wrap.

CHICKEN SALAD

MAKES 1 SERVING

1 rib celery, chopped

1 small carrot, finely chopped

1 tablespoon finely chopped red onion

1 handful fresh parsley, finely chopped

1 handful fresh dill, finely chopped

Juice of ½ lemon

1 tablespoon olive oil or olive oil mayonnaise

Sea salt and freshly ground black pepper to taste

¾ cup chopped cooked chicken (about 5 ounces)

3 cups pre-washed baby arugula

VEGETARIAN OPTION

You can substitute ¾ cup chopped, store-bought marinated tempeh for the chicken. Prepare in the same way.

Combine all the ingredients except the chicken and arugula in a medium bowl and mix thoroughly. Gently fold in the chicken and toss to combine. Serve over arugula.

EASY "TORTILLA" SOUP

....

MAKES 1 SERVING

This zesty soup has all the flavor of traditional Mexican tortilla soup without the refined carbs.

> 2 cups low-sodium chicken broth
> ½ cup cooked chicken, shredded (about 4 ounces)
> ½ cup cooked quinoa (page 253)
> 1 tablespoon finely chopped red onion
> Juice of ½ lime
> Dash hot sauce
> Sea salt and freshly ground black pepper to taste
> 1 tablespoon chopped fresh cilantro
> ¼–½ ripe avocado, cubed

In a small saucepan, combine all the ingredients except the cilantro and avocado. Heat to your desired temperature, then pour into a soup bowl and top with the cilantro and avocado.

GREEN LENTILS WITH SHIITAKE MUSHROOMS

....

MAKES 1 SERVING

Served warm, this scrumptious dish makes for really healthy comfort food. Enjoying it on a cold day feels like a special treat.

> 1 cup green lentils, rinsed and drained
> 2 cups low-sodium vegetable broth
> 4" wakame seaweed *or* 4 pinches shredded
> Leaves of 1 sprig fresh thyme
> Leaves of 1 sprig fresh rosemary, chopped

½ cup parsnips, peeled and sliced into ¼" disks

5 shiitake mushrooms (stems removed), sliced

1 tablespoon tamari

2 cloves garlic, crushed

2 plump scallions, chopped

1 cup watercress, chopped

1½ tablespoons olive oil

¼ teaspoon freshly ground black pepper or to taste

Place the lentils in a pot with the broth and seaweed; bring to a boil. Add the thyme and rosemary leaves, cover, and simmer for 10 minutes. Add the parsnips and mushrooms; cover and simmer for 10 more minutes or until the lentils are tender. Transfer the mixture to a bowl and stir in the remaining ingredients.

MEDITERRANEAN TURKEY LETTUCE WRAP

MAKES 1 SERVING

3 large romaine lettuce leaves

1 rounded tablespoon olive oil mayonnaise

¾ cup roast turkey breast (about 5 ounces), *or* 3–5 slices store-bought turkey breast

1 tablespoon chopped red onion

¼ cup chopped jarred roasted sweet peppers

1 tablespoon chopped fresh parsley

Sea salt and freshly ground black pepper to taste

Arrange the romaine leaves on a plate as if they were bread. Spread olive oil mayonnaise on each leaf. Now build a wrap by placing an equal amount of the turkey, onion, sweet peppers, and parsley on each leaf. Season with salt and pepper, then fold the leaves into a wrap to serve.

PEAR-ARUGULA SALAD WITH CHICKEN & WALNUTS

MAKES 1 SERVING

1 ripe pear, cored and sliced very thin (skin on)

2 tablespoons chopped red onion

½ cup shredded cooked chicken (about 4 ounces)

¼ cup chopped jarred roasted sweet peppers

1 tablespoon raisins

1 tablespoon chopped walnuts

2–3 cups pre-washed arugula

2 tablespoons olive oil

1 tablespoon balsamic vinegar

Sea salt and freshly ground black pepper to taste

Combine the ingredients in a large salad bowl and toss until all components are well dressed.

QUINOA PILAF

MAKES 1 SERVING

½ cup shiitake mushrooms, cleaned, stems removed, and sliced

⅓–½ cup Caramelized Onions (page 266)

1 chicken sausage cut into disks (we like Applegate Farms chicken-apple sausages) *or* ¾ cup cubed roast turkey (about 5 ounces)

¾ cup cooked quinoa (page 253)

½ teaspoon minced fresh sage *or* ¼ teaspoon dried sage

Sea salt and freshly ground black pepper to taste

3 cups washed baby arugula, baby spinach, or watercress

Sauté the mushrooms in the onion mixture until the mushrooms are soft (about 8 minutes). Add the sausage or turkey, cook until heated through, and combine all the ingredients (except the greens) in a large bowl. Serve over arugula or baby spinach—the greens will wilt under the heat of the quinoa.

SOUTHWEST BEAN SALAD

MAKES 1 SERVING

1/3 cup canned chickpeas, rinsed and drained

1/3 cup canned black beans, rinsed and drained

½ cup grape tomatoes, halved

½ medium yellow bell pepper, seeded and diced

2 tablespoons red onion, finely chopped

¼ cup chopped celery

2 teaspoons chopped fresh cilantro

2 tablespoons chopped fresh parsley

1 garlic clove, minced

Pinch ground cumin

Sea salt and freshly ground black pepper to taste

1 tablespoon olive oil

Juice of ½ lime

3 cups pre-washed baby spinach

Combine all the ingredients except the spinach in a bowl and mix well. Spoon over the spinach and serve.

STEAK SALAD WITH TOMATOES & AVOCADO

MAKES 1 SERVING

1 tablespoon olive oil

4 ounces hanger, skirt, or flank steak

2 cups chopped romaine lettuce

1 cup halved cherry tomatoes

¼ ripe avocado, cubed

½ can hearts of palm, drained and cut into ½" disks

½ cup steamed string beans (page 259)

(continued)

Sea salt and freshly ground black pepper to taste

Garlicky Lime Dressing (page 268)

To prepare the steak, heat the olive oil in a skillet over medium-high heat. Season the steak with salt and pepper to taste, then place it in the pan and cook for 5 minutes on each side, or to your desired doneness.

To prepare the salad, combine all the remaining ingredients (except the dressing) in a large bowl and toss. Slice the steak and place it on top of the salad. Top with dressing.

"TACO" SALAD

MAKES 1 SERVING

1 tablespoon olive oil

4 ounces lean, grass-fed ground beef

¼ cup mild salsa

¼ cup canned black beans, rinsed

2 tablespoons chopped red onion

2 tablespoons chopped fresh cilantro

Dash chili powder

Sea salt and freshly ground black pepper to taste

3 cups shredded romaine lettuce

> ### KITCHEN DIVA TIP
> Whenever you're using pre-prepared salsa, make sure that it's made with sea salt.

Heat the olive oil in a skillet over medium heat. Add the beef and brown until cooked through. Drain off any fat, and set aside.

In a medium bowl, combine all the remaining ingredients. Add the beef and toss.

TURKEY BURGERS

. . . .

MAKES 1 SERVING

These yummy burgers are good enough to eat without a bun or regular burger toppings like ketchup, and make a wonderfully healthy option for cookouts.

1 dash garlic powder

¼ teaspoon each: sage, onion powder, no-salt all-purpose seasoning, poultry seasoning

Dash cayenne pepper

Pinch sea salt

Freshly ground black pepper to taste

1 rounded teaspoon 100% fruit peach preserves

1 teaspoon Dijon mustard

½ pound ground, white-meat turkey

2 teaspoons butter

In a small bowl, combine all ingredients except the turkey and butter and mix well. Place the turkey in a medium bowl and fold in the spice mixture, being careful not to overwork the meat. Divide the mixture into two burgers, approximately ¾ inch thick.

In a large skillet, melt the butter over medium-high heat. Add the burgers and cook for 4 minutes on each side or until completely cooked through.

TURKEY EGGPLANT NAPOLEON

. . . .

MAKES 1 SERVING

4 slices medium to large eggplant, peeled and sliced ¼–½" thick

5 ounces ground turkey

1 tablespoon olive oil

¼ cup tomato sauce (we like Muir Glen's crushed tomatoes with basil)

1 clove garlic, grated

(continued)

1 tablespoon chopped fresh basil, plus 4–6 whole
leaves for garnish (optional)
Sea salt and freshly ground black pepper to taste
Pinch red pepper flakes (optional)

Preheat the oven to 375°. Place the eggplant slices on a
cookie sheet lined with parchment paper. Bake in the
oven until tender, about 20 to 30 minutes, flipping
halfway through.

In a medium skillet, sauté the turkey in the olive oil until
it's browned (about 5 minutes). Add the tomato sauce,
garlic, basil, salt and pepper, and red pepper flakes, if
desired; cook for an additional 4 minutes. Remove from
the heat.

Place one slice of the eggplant on a plate and spoon
some of the turkey mixture on top. Then place a second
slice of the eggplant on top of the first and top with
turkey mixture and fresh pepper. Repeat with the
remaining slices and turkey mixture so that you end up
with two napoleons. Top with fresh basil leaves.

KITCHEN DIVA TIP

To remove the bitterness
from the eggplant, sprinkle
each slice lightly with sea
salt (about 1 pinch of salt
in total) and set aside in
a medium bowl. Allow
the slices to sit for 20 to
30 minutes. This will yield
a brownish liquid, which
contains the enzymes that
make the eggplant bitter.
Simply rinse the eggplant
and pat dry with a paper
towel before you begin
cooking.

WILD SALMON SALAD

MAKES 1 SERVING

*For this delicious salad, we use canned wild salmon with the skin and bones
incorporated. You won't taste them, but they will give you an unbelievable hit of
nutrients, along with glowing skin, thanks to the collagen and omega-3s. This salad
also works great served with crackers at a cocktail party. For the faint of heart: You
can use the regular skinless, boneless variety of canned salmon, but the salad will be
drier and nowhere near as yummy.*

1 can (7.5 ounces) wild salmon *with* skin and bones, drained and mashed so
bones and skin are incorporated

1 handful fresh cilantro, washed, dried, and minced

2 scallions, finely chopped

4 ribs celery, finely diced

3 cups pre-washed shredded romaine lettuce

For the dressing:

2 teaspoons lime juice

2 teaspoons olive oil

2 tablespoons Dijon mustard

Sea salt to taste

Freshly ground black pepper to taste

1 generous teaspoon raw honey

In a large bowl, combine the salmon, cilantro, scallions, and celery. Mix and set aside.

To prepare the dressing, whisk all ingredients together in a bowl. Pour over the salmon mixture and toss. Serve over romaine lettuce.

DINNERS

AROMATIC LAMB WITH VEGETABLES

MAKES 2 SERVINGS

1 pound ground lamb

2 cloves garlic, minced

2 teaspoons grated fresh ginger

1 tablespoon chopped cilantro

1 tablespoon chopped fresh mint

½ teaspoon ground cumin

¼ teaspoon ground coriander

¼ teaspoon ground cinnamon

(continued)

½ teaspoon celery seeds

Sea salt and freshly ground black pepper to taste

Juice from ½ lemon

1 tablespoon olive oil

1 tablespoon butter

¾ cup chopped scallions

¾ cup chopped sweet or yellow onions

½ can (14 ounces) crushed tomatoes

½ cup sliced white button mushrooms

½ cup portobello mushrooms, gills removed, sliced

1 package (about 10 ounces) pre-washed baby spinach

> ### KITCHEN DIVA TIP
> You can substitute 1 pound ground turkey, chicken, or grass-fed beef for the lamb.

In a glass bowl, combine the lamb, garlic, ginger, herbs, spices, salt, and lemon juice. Cover and refrigerate for at least half an hour. Heat the oil and butter in a large sauté pan and brown the lamb on medium-high heat, stirring frequently, about 5 minutes. Add all vegetables except for the spinach and cook until tender. Turn the heat down to low, add the spinach, and cover until the spinach wilts, about 2 minutes. Stir to combine the spinach. Serve over quinoa or with baked sweet potato.

BAKED TILAPIA

MAKES 2 SERVINGS

This recipe works equally well with any other light, white, flaky fish, such as sole, flounder, or turbot.

1 pound tilapia fillets

¼ cup lemon juice

½ teaspoon each: thyme, rosemary, paprika

1 tablespoon olive oil or butter

Sea salt and freshly ground black pepper to taste

1 tablespoon chopped fresh parsley

Preheat the oven to 350°. Place the fish in a large casserole dish and pour the lemon juice over the top. Sprinkle with thyme, rosemary, and paprika, and then dot with butter or drizzle with oil. Cook until the flesh is opaque, about 8 to 10 minutes. Sprinkle with parsley and serve over steamed greens—kale and spinach work best.

BBQ CHICKEN V₿

MAKES 2 SERVINGS

This dish requires a bit of advance preparation to marinate the chicken, but the end result is well worth it. The sweet and tangy sauce will be a hit at any BBQ.

1 small onion, chopped fine

2 teaspoons butter

Zest of ½ lime

1 clove garlic, minced

Juice of 2 limes

¾ cup crushed tomatoes

2 teaspoons tomato paste

2 tablespoons balsamic vinegar

2 tablespoons raw honey

2 dashes hot sauce (or to taste)

2 teaspoons brown mustard

Sea salt and freshly ground black pepper to taste

2 boneless, skinless chicken breast halves, pounded thin (about 1 pound)

VEGETARIAN OPTION

You can substitute one 7-ounce package firm tofu cut into cubes for the chicken. The preparation is the same, except you only need to marinate the tofu for 20 minutes before cooking.

In a medium saucepan with a lid, sauté the onion in the butter over a medium-high flame until translucent. Add the lime zest and garlic and sauté for 2 more minutes. Add all the other ingredients, except the chicken, and bring to a boil. Reduce the heat to low and simmer for 20 minutes. Set the sauce aside and allow to cool. Once the sauce has come to room temperature, pour it over the chicken, and let this marinate in the refrigerator for at least 3 hours. Grill the chicken or cook in a nonstick pan for about 5 minutes on each side.

BEEF & QUINOA STUFFED PEPPERS

. . . .

MAKES 2 SERVINGS

This simple dish makes a lovely presentation, and is the perfect choice if you're cooking for company. Instead of using store-bought Worcestershire sauce, which is loaded with sodium and artificial ingredients, we use anchovies and tamari to provide the same kind of kick and impart a wonderful depth of flavor.

1 pound 85–90% lean ground beef (chuck or sirloin)

4 medium-size green, red, orange, or yellow bell peppers

½ cup cooked quinoa (page 253)

1 can (15 ounces) tomato sauce, divided

1 tablespoon tamari

2 cloves garlic, grated

¼ cup finely chopped yellow onion

2 anchovies, mashed into a paste

Sea salt and freshly ground black pepper to taste

1 teaspoon Italian seasoning

1 tablespoon chopped fresh parsley, for garnish

> ### VEGETARIAN OPTION
> . . . .
> You can substitute 1 pound chopped tempeh for the beef. Preparation is the same, except that you should brown the tempeh in 1 tablespoon olive oil and include 1 dash hot sauce and 1 rounded teaspoon ground kelp instead of the anchovy paste.

Preheat the oven to 350°. In a skillet over medium heat, cook the beef until it's evenly browned, and then season with a pinch of sea salt.

Remove and discard the tops, seeds, and membranes of the bell peppers. Arrange the peppers in a baking dish with the hollowed sides facing upward. (Slice the bottoms of the peppers if necessary so that they will stand upright.)

In a bowl, mix the browned beef, cooked quinoa, half of the tomato sauce, tamari, garlic, onion, anchovy paste, sea salt, and pepper. Spoon an equal amount of the mixture into each hollowed pepper. Mix the remaining tomato sauce and Italian seasoning in a bowl, and pour over the stuffed peppers.

Bake 1 hour in the preheated oven or until the peppers are tender.

BRAISED CHICKEN WITH BLACK CHERRY SHALLOT SAUCE

. . . .

MAKES 2 SERVINGS

Black cherry concentrate is packed with inflammation-fighting flavonoids; you can find it in most health food stores near the bottled juices.

2 bone-in chicken breast halves, skin on (about 1½ pounds)

1 plump shallot, minced

1 tablespoon olive oil

½ cup low-sodium chicken broth, plus more as needed

¼ cup mild salsa

3 tablespoons black cherry concentrate

A generous dash each: chili powder, oregano, paprika, cumin, ground cloves, marjoram

Sea salt and freshly ground black pepper to taste

Rinse the chicken in cold water and towel dry; set aside. In a large, deep skillet (with a lid), sauté the shallot in the olive oil on high heat, stirring frequently, until soft, about 3 minutes. Lower the heat to medium and place the chicken in the pan. Add the broth, salsa, and cherry concentrate. Season with salt, pepper, and additional spices to taste; cook the chicken for 5 minutes on each side, adding more broth as needed. Reduce the heat to low, cover with the lid, and continue to simmer until the chicken is cooked through and the juices run clear, about 15 to 20 minutes. If desired, remove the chicken from the pan and cook the sauce longer to reduce.

CITRUS SHRIMP

. . . .

MAKES 2 SERVINGS

Juice of 1 lemon

Juice of 1 lime

¼ cup orange juice (optional)

(continued)

1 clove garlic, crushed

¼ teaspoon red pepper flakes

1 tablespoon olive oil

½ cup chopped fresh parsley

8 ounces shrimp, peeled and de-veined (about 14 medium shrimp)

½ cup mild salsa

½ avocado

Preheat the oven to broil. Combine the lemon juice, lime juice, orange juice, garlic, red pepper, olive oil, and parsley in a bowl and whisk together. Place the shrimp in the mixture and marinate in the refrigerator for at least 30 minutes.

Remove the shrimp from the bowl and discard the extra marinade. Line a pan with foil and broil the shrimp in the oven for about 5 minutes, or until they just begin to turn pink. Serve topped with salsa and avocado.

CUBAN CHICKEN V
....

MAKES 2 SERVINGS

1 pound boneless, skinless chicken thighs

1 clove garlic, peeled and crushed

½ teaspoon ground cumin

1 lemon, sliced, seeds removed

½ cup fresh lime juice

½ cup orange juice

½ large sweet or yellow onion, cut into thin rings

2 tablespoons olive oil for marinade, plus 1 teaspoon for cooking

Sea salt and freshly ground black pepper to taste

½ red bell pepper, finely chopped

1 container (10 ounces) pre-washed arugula

Rinse and paper-towel-dry the chicken thighs. Set aside. In a large glass bowl, combine all the ingredients (except the red pepper and arugula) and mix to form the marinade. Add the chicken and marinate in the refrigerator for at least 3 hours.

Remove the chicken, lemons, and onions from the marinade; discard the lemons. Heat the remaining teaspoon of olive oil in a sauté pan over medium-high heat and sauté the peppers and marinated onions until soft, about 4 to 5 minutes. Set aside. Brown the chicken over medium-high heat in the same pan as the peppers with the remaining olive oil until a crust forms on the outside and the chicken is completely cooked through, about 4 minutes on each side. Put the remaining marinade in a small saucepan and bring to a boil. Reduce the heat and simmer until the liquid has reduced by half, approximately 5 minutes. Add the peppers, onion, and chicken, cover with the lid, and simmer for 2 minutes. Serve over raw baby arugula.

> ## VEGETARIAN OPTION
>
> You can substitute one 7-ounce package firm tofu cut into cubes for the chicken. Preparation is the same, except you should marinate the tofu for only 20 minutes.

GINGER SHRIMP & CABBAGE STIR-FRY

MAKES 2 SERVINGS

2 tablespoons olive oil

1 medium sweet or yellow onion, chopped

4 cloves garlic, chopped

8 ounces shrimp, peeled and de-veined (about 14 medium shrimp), *or* 1 pound chicken breast or beef, sliced into thin strips

1 stalk broccoli—peel stem and chop; reserve flowers

½ head green cabbage (approximately 1 pound), shredded

4 medium carrots, grated fine

1 medium zucchini, chopped

Water

1" piece fresh ginger, grated

2 leaves kale or collards, de-veined and chopped

1 teaspoon toasted sesame oil

(continued)

1 teaspoon tamari (plus more to taste)
1 teaspoon brown rice vinegar
2 teaspoons mirin

> ### VEGETARIAN OPTION
> ....
> You can substitute one 7-ounce package firm tofu cut into cubes for the shrimp.

Place a large skillet on a high flame. Add the olive oil, onion, and garlic, and sauté until transparent (about 10 minutes). Add the shrimp and cook until done and pink (about 5 minutes; if using chicken, the strips should be cooked through until the juices run clear; if using beef, simply cook to desired doneness). Add the broccoli stem, cabbage, carrots, and zucchini, lower the flame to medium, add a splash of water, and cook 5 minutes. Add the ginger, kale, and broccoli flowers; cook 3 minutes. Add the sesame oil, tamari, and brown rice vinegar, stirring frequently. Serve over brown rice.

GRILLED GRASS-FED LONDON BROIL
....

MAKES 2 SERVINGS

Used as a marinade, black cherry concentrate—which is high in flavonoids—makes steak healthier because it reduces free radicals.

4 garlic cloves, chopped
½ bunch fresh parsley, chopped
2 tablespoons tamari
2 tablespoons black cherry concentrate
Leaves of 3 sprigs fresh rosemary, finely chopped
Sea salt and freshly ground black pepper to taste
1 tablespoon olive oil, plus 1 teaspoon more for cooking
12 ounces grass-fed London broil or sirloin steak

Blend all the ingredients except the steak in a food processor until combined and smooth. Put the steak in a bowl and coat with the mixture. Place in the refrigerator and marinate for at least 30 minutes. Place a grill or sauté pan over medium-high heat and coat with oil. Cook the steak on medium heat about 5 minutes on each side, or to your desired doneness. Remove from the pan and allow the steak to rest about 5 minutes before cutting.

HERBED MAPLE CHICKEN

MAKES 2 SERVINGS

Don't be afraid of chicken skin! Though it's been long vilified by dieters, new research shows that 55 percent of the fats in chicken skin are actually monounsaturated—the heart-healthy kind—and that a chicken breast with the skin still on has just fifty calories more than a plain one. So forget about the fat and savor the gloriously crisp skin in this recipe and others.

    2 tablespoons olive oil
    Juice of 1 lemon or lime
    1 tablespoon brown mustard
    1 tablespoon grade B maple syrup
    1 generous dash each: paprika, oregano, chili powder, sage
    1 handful fresh parsley, chopped fine
    Leaves of 2 sprigs fresh thyme
    ½ small yellow onion, minced
    2 cloves garlic, minced fine
    Sea salt to taste (about 2 generous pinches)
    2 bone-in chicken breast halves, skin on (about 1½ pounds)

Preheat the oven to 375°. Place all the ingredients except the chicken in a large bowl and mix well. Place the chicken in the bowl and cover with the spice mixture. At this point, you can either marinate the chicken in the refrigerator (anywhere from 30 minutes to overnight) or go ahead and place the chicken in a glass casserole dish, skin-side down, cover with foil, and bake for 20 minutes. Then remove the foil, turn the chicken over, baste with juices, and continue to bake uncovered for another 20 minutes, or until the juices run clear. Serve over brown rice or quinoa.

HERBED SALMON ⓥ

MAKES 2 SERVINGS

    2 fillets (6 ounces each) wild salmon or arctic char
    2 tablespoons olive oil, divided
    1 tablespoon freshly squeezed lime juice
    1 tablespoon chopped shallots
    1 teaspoon chopped fresh dill
    ¼ cup finely chopped red or yellow bell pepper
    Dash cayenne pepper
    Sea salt and freshly ground black pepper to taste

> ### VEGETARIAN OPTION
>
> You can substitute one 12-ounce package of tempeh for the fish. Preparation is the same, except that you should bake the tempeh for 30 to 40 minutes and serve topped with ¼ cup Caramelized Onions (page 266).

Preheat the oven to 350°. Place the fish in a large casserole dish and drizzle with 1½ tablespoons of the olive oil. Add the lime juice and then turn the fish to marinate on both sides. In a separate bowl, combine the shallots, dill, bell pepper, cayenne, sea salt and pepper, and remaining olive oil. Cover the fish with mixture. Cover loosely with baking foil and bake for 8 to 12 minutes, or until the flesh is opaque.

LEMON SNAPPER

MAKES 2 SERVINGS

    2 tablespoons lemon juice
    1 teaspoon lemon zest
    1 tablespoon butter, melted
    Sea salt and freshly ground black pepper to taste
    Pinch nutmeg
    1 pound red snapper
    Lemon wedges, for garnish

Preheat the oven to 350°. Combine the lemon juice, lemon zest, butter, salt, pepper, and nutmeg in a small bowl. Place the fish in a glass casserole dish and spoon the mixture over. Bake uncovered for about 15 minutes, or until the flesh is opaque. Garnish with lemon wedges.

ROAST TURKEY THIGH

MAKES 2 SERVINGS

1 pound boneless turkey thigh, skin on

1 clove garlic, minced

1 teaspoon Dijon mustard

1 teaspoon chopped fresh rosemary leaves

½ teaspoon sage

½ teaspoon chopped fresh thyme leaves

½ teaspoon onion powder

½ teaspoon paprika

Sea salt and freshly ground black pepper to taste

1 tablespoon olive oil

1 tablespoon butter

1 tablespoon freshly squeezed lemon juice

1 cup low-sodium vegetable broth

Preheat the oven to 325°. Place the turkey, skin-side up, on a rack in a roasting pan or in a casserole dish. In a small bowl, combine the garlic, mustard, spices, salt, pepper, olive oil, butter, and lemon juice to make a paste. Loosen the turkey skin and rub half of the mixture directly on the meat. Spread the remaining paste evenly on the skin. Pour the broth into the bottom of the roasting pan.

Cover the turkey with foil and roast for 25 minutes. Then remove the foil and cook for an additional 10 minutes or until a meat thermometer reads 165° when inserted into the thickest part of the meat. When the turkey is done, remove from the oven, cover with foil, and allow it to rest at room temperature for 15 minutes. Slice and serve with the pan juices spooned over the turkey.

TURKEY CURRY
....

MAKES 2 SERVINGS

1 onion, thinly sliced (about 1 cup)

3 cloves garlic, finely chopped

2 teaspoons olive oil

2 teaspoons butter

12 ounces skinless, boneless turkey breast, cut into cubes

1 cup canned, diced tomatoes

1 cup canned chickpeas, rinsed and drained

¼ cup raisins

1 rounded tablespoon curry powder

¼ teaspoon turmeric

Dash cardamom

1 teaspoon grated fresh ginger

Pinch sea salt

Freshly ground black pepper to taste

Dash cayenne pepper

½ cup low-sodium chicken broth

½ cup light coconut milk

In a large pot, sauté the onion and garlic in oil and butter until translucent. Add the turkey and sear on all sides. Add tomatoes, chickpeas, raisins, curry, turmeric, cardamom, and ginger, and then season with salt, pepper, and cayenne to taste. Add the chicken broth and coconut milk and bring to a boil. Reduce the heat and simmer until the turkey is cooked through, about 15 to 20 minutes. Serve over brown rice or quinoa.

VEGETABLES & SIDES

BAKED SWEET POTATO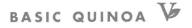

MAKES 2 SERVINGS

1 large *or* 2 small sweet potatoes (yams, garnet yams or Japanese sweet
   potatoes work, too!)
2 teaspoons olive oil
Sea salt to taste

Preheat the oven to 400°. Pierce the potatoes with a fork all over to vent. Lay the
potatoes on a cookie sheet, rub with oil, and sprinkle with salt. Bake for about 20
minutes then turn over and bake for another 20 minutes until totally soft and the skin
has crisped.

BASIC QUINOA

MAKES 2 SERVINGS

*We recommend that you double or even triple this recipe and use the leftovers in
your other recipes throughout the week. Soaking the quinoa ahead of time helps it
to cook evenly and loosens up the outer coating of saponin, a naturally occurring
herbicide that can give a bitter taste if not removed. Adding the butter gives the
quinoa a nice creaminess and provides a dose of healthy fats and omega-3s.*

1 cup quinoa
2 cups cold water or low-sodium chicken broth
Sea salt to taste
1 tablespoon butter

In a large bowl, soak the quinoa for 15 to 30 minutes in enough filtered water to
cover. Strain the quinoa using a mesh strainer, rinse again with cool water, and then
transfer to a medium-size pot with a lid. Add water or broth. Bring to a boil, add salt,

(continued)

cover with the lid, lower the heat, and simmer for 12 to 15 minutes or until all the water is absorbed. Remove the quinoa from the heat and let it stand for 5 minutes with the lid on. Fluff gently with a fork and add the butter.

GARLICKY LIME SALAD 🅥

MAKES 1 SERVING

This yummy salad is one of our favorites. On its own, it can be used as a side for meats and fish, and when topped with protein it makes a terrific stand-alone lunch. Try our different protein suggestions below and see which you like best.

> 3 cups salad greens (arugula, baby spinach, Bibb or red-leaf lettuce, or mesclun)
> ½ pear, cored and diced (skin on)
> 2 tablespoons chopped walnuts
> Garlicky Lime Dressing (page 268)

In a large bowl, mix the greens, pear, and walnuts. Add your desired amount of dressing.

KITCHEN DIVA TIP

For a lunch salad, add one of the following options:
- 1–2 hard-boiled eggs, sliced and served on top
- ¾ cup (about 5 ounces) roast turkey breast, shredded
- 1 can (3.75 ounces) skinless, boneless sardines packed in olive oil

KALE CHIPS

MAKES 2–4 SERVINGS

High in nutrients and low in calories, kale chips are essentially a free food—you can eat as many of these tasty chips as you want, which is a good thing since they are tough to put down.

1 bunch kale, stems removed and torn into 1" pieces
1 tablespoon olive oil
Pinch sea salt

Preheat the oven to 350°. In a bowl, toss the kale well with oil and sea salt, making sure that the pieces are evenly covered. Place the kale on a baking sheet lined with parchment paper. Bake until the edges are browned but not burned, turning once, about 10 to 15 minutes. You will need to watch them closely, as they cook fast.

PUMPKIN-QUINOA RISOTTO

MAKES 2 SERVINGS

This dish is so good that it's like a naughty treat. You can even enjoy it as a vegetarian entrée with a salad on the side.

2 tablespoons canned pumpkin (*not* pumpkin pie filling)
Low-sodium chicken or vegetable broth as needed
1 tablespoon butter ,
1 cup cooked quinoa (page 253)
Sea salt and freshly ground black pepper to taste
¼ cup Caramelized Onions (page 266)

In a medium saucepan over medium heat, thin out the canned pumpkin with a few tablespoons of chicken broth. Add the butter and stir to create a glistening sauce. Fold in the cooked quinoa. Season with salt and pepper and top with Caramelized Onions.

PUMPKIN-RAISIN COLLARD GREENS

MAKES 2 SERVINGS

1 bunch collard greens, washed, stems separated
    from leaves; chop both

2 teaspoons tamari

2 teaspoons toasted sesame oil

¼ cup Toasted Pumpkin Seeds (page 271)

1 handful raisins

> ### KITCHEN DIVA TIP
>
> You can switch out the pumpkin seeds for walnuts or almonds; tamari for sea salt; or the toasted sesame oil for olive oil.

Place the collard stems in a steamer with an inch of water. Bring to a boil, then cover and steam for about 2 minutes or until the stems become a vibrant green color. Toss in the leaves and cover for 3 to 4 more minutes, until the leaves are limp and tender. Using tongs, transfer the greens into a large bowl. Add the tamari first, then the sesame oil, pumpkin seeds, and raisins. Mix well.

ROASTED BUTTERNUT SQUASH

MAKES 2 SERVINGS

1 small butternut squash, sliced in half, seeds removed

1 tablespoon olive oil

Sea salt and freshly ground black pepper to taste

> ### KITCHEN DIVA TIP
>
> To satisfy a sweet tooth, drizzle 1 teaspoon grade B maple syrup over the flesh side before serving. You can sprinkle with cinnamon as well.

Preheat the oven to 375°. Drizzle the squash on both sides with olive oil, sprinkle with salt and pepper, and place on a cookie sheet, flesh-side down. Roast for 30 to 50 minutes, depending on size, or until you can easily pierce the skin with a fork.

ROASTED CAULIFLOWER ⱱ

MAKES 2 SERVINGS

4 cups roughly chopped cauliflower

2 tablespoons olive oil

Leaves of 3 sprigs fresh thyme, chopped

1 garlic clove, chopped

Juice of ½ lemon

Sea salt and freshly ground black pepper to taste

Preheat the oven to 375°. Spread the cauliflower in an even layer on a large, rimmed baking sheet. In a bowl, whisk together the olive oil, spices, and lemon juice until combined, and pour over the cauliflower. Roast in the oven until fork-tender and golden brown, about 20 to 25 minutes, turning once halfway through.

KITCHEN DIVA TIP

Mashed cauliflower is equally tasty and nutrient-packed: Simply prepare as above, omitting the lemon juice and halving the olive oil. Cook 25 minutes or until golden brown, then puree to a mashed potato consistency and finish with 1 tablespoon butter.

MISO-SESAME SALAD ⱱ

MAKES 2 SERVINGS

3 cups pre-washed baby spinach

1 cup cherry tomatoes, halved

2 tablespoons Miso-Sesame Dressing (page 269)

Combine the ingredients in a large bowl and top with the dressing.

SIMPLE STEAMED GREENS ⅤG

MAKES 2 SERVINGS

This recipe works equally well for any of the powerhouse greens: kale, collard greens, Swiss chard, rainbow chard, or red chard. When cooking kale, we like Tuscan kale (also known as Lacinato kale or Dinosaur kale because of the leaves' bumpy texture) because you don't have to remove the stems. If you use curly- or flat-leaf kale, you will need to remove the stems and either discard them or cook them separately (see the Kitchen Diva Tip, below). With chard, you can leave the stems on as well.

2 cups roughly chopped kale (or other greens)
Water

Place about 2 inches of water in the bottom of a pot and bring to a boil. Place the kale in a steamer basket, cover with a lid, and cook on medium-high until the kale is limp and tender and a bright green color, about 4 minutes.

KITCHEN DIVA TIPS

- With curly- or flat-leaf kale and collard greens, you can eat the stems, too, if you prepare them right: Simply remove and chop the stems, then steam them in your steamer basket for 2 minutes before adding the leaves.
- For another dimension of flavor, substitute chicken broth for the water, or add either 1 clove grated garlic or a ¼-inch disk of fresh, peeled ginger to the pot when you add the leaves.
- You can also top your greens with any of the following: a dash of tamari, 1 teaspoon toasted sesame oil, 1 teaspoon olive oil, or 1 tablespoon melted butter. Or toss them with any powdered spice that calls to you.

SIMPLE STEAMED VEGETABLES

MAKES 2 SERVINGS

We prefer to steam our vegetables since they retain more flavor and nutrients that way. You can use the directions and cooking times below to prepare a variety of delicious sides.

2 cups of any vegetable you like
1 tablespoon butter
Sea salt to taste

Place about 2 inches of water in the bottom of a pot and bring to a boil. Place the vegetables in a steamer basket, cover with a lid, and cook on medium-high until they are slightly tender but not mushy or overcooked.

KITCHEN DIVA TIP

How long to steam your veggies:

- Asparagus: 8–10 minutes
- Broccoli: 8–10 minutes
- Cauliflower: 8–15 minutes
- Carrots: 4–5 minutes if slices, 10–15 minutes if whole
- Snap peas: 3–5 minutes
- String beans: 5–15 minutes
- Zucchini, sliced: 5–10 minutes

SPINACH SALAD WITH HONEY MUSTARD DRESSING

MAKES 2 SERVINGS

3 cups pre-washed baby spinach
1 apple, cored and chopped (skin on)
¼ cup sliced Toasted Almonds (page 270)
2 tablespoons Honey Mustard Dressing (page 268)

Combine the spinach, apple, and almonds in a bowl and mix well. Top with dressing and serve.

TOMATO-CUCUMBER SALAD V𝕓

MAKES 2 SERVINGS

 1 cup cherry tomatoes, halved

 ½ cup cucumber, chopped

 ¼ cup chopped red onion

 ¼ cup chopped fresh parsley

 1 teaspoon olive oil

 1 teaspoon red wine vinegar

 Sea salt and freshly ground black pepper to taste

Combine all the ingredients in a bowl and mix well.

DESSERTS

BAKED APPLES V𝕓

MAKES 2 SERVINGS

 2 medium to large apples, cores removed (skin on)

 Handful raisins

 ¼ cup chopped pecans or slivered Toasted Almonds (page 270)

 1 tablespoon black cherry concentrate or grade B maple syrup

 Cinnamon and ground cloves to taste

 1 tablespoon butter

 ½ cup water

KITCHEN DIVA TIP

You can also try adding ginger or nutmeg to this dish.

Preheat the oven to 375°. Slice the very bottom off the apples so they sit upright in a glass casserole dish. Place the raisins, nuts, and syrup in center of each apple, sprinkle with spices, and dot with butter. Pour the water into the bottom of the dish. Place in the oven and baste every 20 minutes until fork-tender, about 40 minutes to 1 hour. You will also notice that the skin will split—this is a sign that the apples are done.

BAKED BANANAS WITH VANILLA-MAPLE SYRUP

MAKES 2 SERVINGS

    1 teaspoon grade B maple syrup
    ½ teaspoon vanilla extract
    2 ripe medium bananas, peeled and halved lengthwise
    1 teaspoon butter
    1 dash cinnamon
    1 dash cocoa powder
    ¼ cup chopped pecans

Preheat the oven to 375°. Combine the maple syrup and vanilla in a small bowl. Place the bananas on a greased cookie sheet, dot with butter, drizzle with the vanilla-maple syrup, and sprinkle with cinnamon. Bake for 8 minutes, then turn over and bake another 8 minutes or until the bananas are caramelized. Dust with cocoa powder and top with pecans.

BANANA SMOOTHIE

MAKES 2 SERVINGS

This recipe works best when the bananas are freckled and very ripe. The additional sweetness you get from the extra ripening will really satisfy your sweet tooth. If crushed ice is readily available, use crushed ice to make the preparation easier.

    3 cups ice
    3 cups unsweetened almond milk
    2 teaspoons vanilla extract
    2 very ripe bananas, peeled, cut into ½" slices, and frozen
    2 tablespoons grade B maple syrup
    2 pinches sea salt (optional)

Place all the ingredients in a food processor or blender and blend until smooth and frothy.

KITCHEN DIVA TIP

For more smoothie variations, see page 274.

BLUEBERRY SORBET

MAKES 2 SERVINGS

This recipe works best in a food processor, but you can use a blender or immersion blender as well. The honey will freeze to form a ribbon that adds a sudden burst of sweetness whenever you encounter it.

1 bag (8 ounces) frozen blueberries
1 tablespoon raw honey

Thaw the blueberries for 10 to 15 minutes; the berries should still be frozen, but able to move freely in a food processor. Place the berries and honey in the food processor and pulse until blended.

KITCHEN DIVA TIPS

- For another layer of flavor, add 1 teaspoon chopped fresh mint to the blueberries before blending.
- To make a peach sorbet, use 1 bag frozen peaches instead.
- This sorbet will solidify if refrozen; you can use that to your advantage by using any leftovers to make popsicles—a perfect low-cal snack. You can find plastic popsicle molds in cute shapes online or at any Kmart or Target.

CRUSTLESS CHERRY PIE

MAKES 2–4 SERVINGS

1 bag (8 ounces) frozen cherries

¼ cup apple juice

Juice of ½ lemon

Thaw the cherries and strain to remove excess liquid. Preheat the oven to 375°. Place all the ingredients in a glass casserole dish and bake for about 30 minutes.

KITCHEN DIVA TIP

Any leftovers from this yummy dessert can also be used as a breakfast compote—try spooning 1 tablespoon over your Basic Oats (page 226) or Vanilla Oatmeal with Raisins (page 231) in the morning. You can also use it as a dressing for chicken or turkey breasts and wraps.

CHILLED HONEYDEW SOUP

MAKES 2 SERVINGS

This recipe works best when the honeydew is ripe to slightly overripe. To choose a ripe honeydew, simply smell the melon—if it's not really fragrant, it's not ripe. You can also ripen a melon at home in your kitchen by allowing it to stand unrefrigerated for several days.

½ large, ripe honeydew, cut into 1" pieces

Juice of 1 lime

1 tablespoon finely chopped fresh mint

¼ cup full-fat Greek yogurt

Place the honeydew and lime juice in a food processor and blend until smooth. In a separate bowl, combine the mint and yogurt and mix well. Ladle the soup into two bowls and top with the mint-yogurt mixture.

CHOCOLATE-COVERED STRAWBERRIES

. . . .

MAKES 2 SERVINGS

    2 cups fresh strawberries, halved, stems removed
    1 tablespoon cocoa powder

Place the strawberries and cocoa powder together in a ziplock bag or container with a cover. Shake to coat the strawberries evenly with the cocoa.

COCOA-DIPPED BANANA WITH TOASTED COCONUT

. . . .

MAKES 2 SERVINGS

    2 bananas
    6 tablespoons Cocoa Cream (page 267)
    2 tablespoons Toasted Coconut (page 271)
    1 teaspoon cocoa powder (for dusting; optional)

Cut the bananas in half lengthwise and then in half again. Spread Cocoa Cream on each piece. Place the coconut in a small dish and dip the cream side of the bananas in the coconut to coat. You can dust with cocoa powder to garnish.

ORANGE SHERBET

. . . .

MAKES 2 SERVINGS

    1¾ cups orange juice
    1 cup coconut water for blending

Pour the orange juice into an ice cube tray and freeze overnight. Transfer the frozen cubes to a food processor or blender, add the coconut water, and pulse until smooth.

RASPBERRY MELON PARFAIT ⅴ̶

MAKES 2 SERVINGS

This dish makes a lovely presentation. If it looks big, keep in mind that cantaloupe has very few calories! You can choose a ripe cantaloupe by smelling the melon— if it's not really fragrant, it's not ripe.

1 ripe cantaloupe, cut in half crosswise (*not* lengthwise), seeds removed

1 cup fresh raspberries or blackberries

2 tablespoons Cashew Cream (page 267)

2 teaspoons black cherry concentrate

KITCHEN DIVA TIP

Instead of the raspberries, you can use any other kind of fresh fruit: Diced strawberries, diced peaches, or blueberries all work well.

Cut a thin layer off the bottom of melon so it's stable on a plate. Fill the center of the melon with the raspberries and top with the Cashew Cream. Drizzle black cherry concentrate on top.

VANILLA-SCENTED POACHED PEARS ⅴ̶

MAKES 2 SERVINGS

Most commercial vanillas contain a lot of sugar and chemicals, so for this recipe, try to use organic vanilla extract—make sure you buy the kind that includes alcohol rather than glycerin. Organic vanillas also give desserts a much richer flavor.

2 Bosc pears, skin on

2 cups apple juice

Generous dash: cloves, cinnamon, ground cardamom

1 tablespoon grade B maple syrup

1 teaspoon vanilla extract

Preheat the oven to 375°. Cut the bottoms off the pears so they are stable in a deep glass casserole dish. Pour in the apple juice and sprinkle with spices. Bake until fork-

(continued)

tender, basting every 15 minutes or so; cooking time is about 1 hour. Transfer the pears to a separate dish and pour the remaining juice into a small saucepan. Add the maple syrup and vanilla and bring the liquid to a boil, then lower the heat and simmer until reduced by half. Spoon the sauce over the pears and serve.

WATERMELON REFRESHER Ⅴ

MAKES 2 SERVINGS

Chilling the watermelon to very cold will give this drink a satisfying, icy texture.

> 2 cups chilled, seedless watermelon chunks
> 2 slices cucumber, for garnish

Place the watermelon in the food processor and blend until smooth. Garnish with cucumber on the side.

KITCHEN DIVA TIP

For another layer of flavor, try blending the cucumber slices in with the watermelon rather than simply enjoying them on the side.

DRESSINGS, DIPS, & TOPPINGS

CARAMELIZED ONIONS Ⅴ

MAKES 2 CUPS

These wonderful onions add a sweet and savory kick to many of our dishes. This recipe can be easily doubled for use throughout the week.

> 2 teaspoons butter
> 2 teaspoons olive oil
> 2 cups sliced Vidalia or yellow onions (about 2 large onions)
> Sea salt and freshly ground black pepper to taste
> Low-sodium chicken or vegetable broth as needed, about ¼–½ cup

In a large sauté pan over medium-high heat, melt the butter and the olive oil. Add the onions, salt, and pepper; cook for about 5 to 10 minutes, stirring often. Reduce the heat to low and continue to cook, stirring often and adding a splash of broth as necessary to keep the onions from sticking. When the color changes to a deep golden brown and the onions are wilted and creamy, they are done—about 20 to 30 minutes.

CASHEW CREAM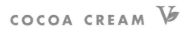

MAKES 2 CUPS

Our Cashew Cream makes a great substitute for mayonnaise and provides a dose of protein and the healthy fats your body needs. It also works as a yummy spread for crackers and a dip for vegetables.

- 1 cup raw cashews
- ¾ cup filtered water

In a food processor, pulse the nuts until they are finely ground. Slowly add the water to your desired texture: less water for thicker "cream," more for thinner.

COCOA CREAM

MAKES ¾ CUP

In this recipe, we add cocoa powder to our Cashew Cream to make our very own version of Nutella—a perfect, healthy snack when combined with any fruit.

- ½ cup Cashew Cream (page 267)
- 2 teaspoons cocoa powder
- 2 teaspoons grade B maple syrup

Combine all the ingredients in a small bowl and mix well. Serve over any fruit: Bananas, strawberries, and apple slices all work well.

also or misleading statement #notscience

DAIKON RADISH RELISH

MAKES ¾ CUP

Daikon radish is one of the few vegetables known to actually <u>boost your metabolism</u>. This relish makes a good pairing with any of our fish recipes, including Lemon Snapper (page 250) and Baked Tilapia (page 242).

    1 daikon radish (about 10" long)
    1 teaspoon tamari
    2 teaspoons toasted sesame oil

Grate the daikon into a medium bowl. Add the tamari and toasted sesame oil; stir to combine.

GARLICKY LIME DRESSING

MAKES 1 CUP

    1 garlic clove, crushed and minced
    ½ cup olive oil
    ¼ cup fresh lime juice
    2 tablespoons raw honey
    2 tablespoons finely chopped red onion
    Sea salt and freshly ground black pepper to taste

Combine all the ingredients in a food processor or blender and pulse until blended.

HONEY MUSTARD DRESSING

MAKES 1¼ CUPS

    ½ cup Dijon mustard
    ¼ cup raw honey
    Juice of ½ lemon

¼ cup olive oil

Generous pinch sea salt

Whisk all the ingredients together in a small bowl and serve.

LEMON GINGER TAHINI SAUCE

MAKES 1½ CUPS

This delicious sauce is the perfect way to liven up just about any vegetable. It's great over broccoli, string beans, or any steamed green; you can use it as a dressing for salads; and a thicker version works as a dip for crudités. Plus, with all that tahini, it's loaded with calcium—most people don't know that sesame seeds actually contain more calcium than milk!

½ bunch fresh parsley, chopped

1 clove garlic, chopped fine

1" fresh ginger, grated

Zest of ½ lemon

2 rounded tablespoons tahini

1 tablespoon tamari

½ cup water

> ### KITCHEN DIVA TIP
>
> To make a thicker dip for crudités, add the water gradually while pulsing until you reach your desired consistency.

Place all the ingredients in a food processor and pulse until blended.

MISO-SESAME DRESSING

MAKES 1 CUP

1 tablespoon cider vinegar

Juice of 1 lemon

1 tablespoon lemon zest

2 tablespoons sweet white miso paste

2 cloves garlic, chopped

2 teaspoons raw honey

½ cup toasted sesame oil

(continued)

Combine all the ingredients except the oil in a food processor and blend on high speed until mixed. With the food processor on medium, slowly add the oil. Water can be added if a thinner consistency is desired.

ONION DIP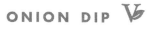

MAKES 1¼ CUPS

    ½ cup Caramelized Onions (page 266)
    ¾ cup Cashew Cream (page 267)
    Sea salt to taste

Combine the onions and Cashew Cream in a food processor or blender and blend until smooth. Season with salt as necessary.

TOASTED ALMONDS

MAKES 2 CUPS

If you buy roasted almonds at the store, you never know what kinds of oils they contain, and they tend to go rancid much more quickly. Still, we love the rich, nutty flavor that roasted almonds impart, so we toast our own. It's incredibly easy to do, and then you can add the almonds to dishes throughout the week.

    2 cups raw sliced almonds

Place the almonds in a stainless-steel skillet and "toast" over medium-high heat, keeping them moving at all times, until they turn golden brown. They will cook very quickly—in only a minute or two—so watch them closely.

TOASTED COCONUT V̄

MAKES 2 CUPS

A delicious source of healthy fats, toasted coconut makes a perfect addition to any dessert.

2 cups loosely packed, shredded unsweetened coconut

Heat a skillet over medium heat. Once the skillet gets warm, add the shredded coconut, spreading it out in a single layer. Cook the coconut, tossing or stirring constantly to prevent burning, until the flakes start to become brown. Transfer to a plate to cool.

> ### KITCHEN DIVA TIP
> To retain flavor and prevent sogginess in your toasted coconut, always store it in an airtight container in a dark, dry place.

TOASTED PUMPKIN SEEDS V̄

MAKES ½ CUP

Raw pumpkin seeds, also known as pepitas, are available in the nuts and seeds section of any health food store. A serving size is considered to be a tablespoon or two; you can sprinkle them over salads or any steamed green, or eat them on their own as a snack.

½ cup raw pumpkin seeds
Sea salt to taste

Sauté the raw pumpkin seeds in a skillet over medium-high heat, stirring often, until they "pop" and become golden brown. Remove from the heat and salt to taste. Store in a glass jar.

BEVERAGES

CITRUS COOLER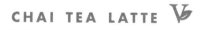

MAKES 6 CUPS

Better than any artificial vitamin water, this refreshing cooler makes it easy to drink water throughout the day. You can use this recipe to make any of the varieties listed below—or invent your own!

6 cups filtered water
1 lime, sliced
1 lemon, sliced
1 orange, sliced

Place the water in a glass pitcher, add the sliced fruit, and refrigerate overnight. Strain the slices through a fine-mesh strainer before drinking.

KITCHEN DIVA TIP

For different flavors, simply add the following instead of the citrus:
- Cucumber Cooler: 1 large cucumber, sliced thin
- Strawberry Cooler: 1 cup diced fresh strawberries, stems removed
- Mint Cooler: 1 cup finely chopped fresh mint

CHAI TEA LATTE

MAKES 1 SERVING

½ cup unsweetened almond milk
1 cup strong black tea or green tea

Dash each: cinnamon, cardamom, ground black pepper, clove, ground fennel, ginger

2 teaspoons honey

Whisk all the ingredients together in a small sauce pot over medium heat until frothy and steamy (do not bring to a boil, or the almond milk will separate). Strain the liquid through a fine-mesh sieve and serve.

HOT CHOCOLATE

MAKES 1 SERVING

1 cup unsweetened almond milk

2 teaspoons grade B maple syrup

1 rounded teaspoon cocoa powder

1 teaspoon vanilla extract

Pinch sea salt (optional)

In a small sauce pot, whisk all the ingredients together over medium heat until frothy and steamy (do not bring to a boil, or the almond milk will separate).

LATTE

MAKES 1 SERVING

1 cup unsweetened almond milk

1 rounded teaspoon instant herbal or grain "coffee"

1 teaspoon honey or grade B maple syrup

Dash cinnamon

Whisk together all the ingredients (except the cinnamon) in a small sauce pot until steamy and frothy (do not bring to a boil, or the almond milk will separate). Remove from the heat and sprinkle with cinnamon.

VANILLA SMOOTHIE 💗

. . . .

MAKES 1 SERVING

We use almond milk instead of cow's milk or yogurt to make our smoothies, so the texture is a bit different: frothy and delicious, but not as thick. But you can enjoy these smoothies guilt-free since a cup of almond milk only has thirty-five calories! Any of the variations below work well for a snack when you are craving something sweet. If crushed ice is readily available, use it to make the preparation easier.

1½ cups ice
1½ cups unsweetened almond milk
1 teaspoon vanilla extract
1 tablespoon grade B maple syrup
Pinch sea salt (optional)

Place all the ingredients in a food processor or blender and blend until smooth and frothy.

KITCHEN DIVA TIP

You can use our Vanilla Smoothie recipe to make any of these additional flavors:
- Chocolate Shake: Add 1½ teaspoons cocoa powder.
- Mochaccino: Prepare the Chocolate Shake version and add 1 teaspoon instant herbal or grain coffee.
- Green Tea: To the Vanilla Smoothie recipe, add ½ teaspoon powdered green tea (also known as matcha powder).
- Chai: Use ice cubes made from strong black tea, and add a dash of cinnamon, ginger, cardamom, and clove to the Vanilla Smoothie recipe.
- Lemon: Add 1 teaspoon lemon extract in place of the vanilla.
- Coconut: Add 1 teaspoon coconut extract in place of the vanilla.
- Strawberry: Use only 1 cup ice and add ½ cup frozen strawberries.

RESOURCES

Anytime you start a new workout or weight-loss regimen, it can be both fun and helpful to connect with other people who are doing the program, just like you. We invite you to join us on Facebook, where you can share your experiences with other Physique 57 followers and post questions for our instructors: www.facebook.com/physique57.com. For more inspiring client success stories, please visit our website: www.physique57.com. We also invite you to send us your own success story (we love before and after pictures!) to success@physiques57.com.

For playground balls, workout wear, and our complete series of DVDs:
   www.physique57.com

For stylish athletic and yoga wear:
   Lululemon Athletica
   877-263-9300
   www.lululemon.com

For organic food products:
   Diamond Organics (offers overnight home delivery)
   888-ORGANIC
   www.diamondorganics.com

Trader Joe's
   www.traderjoes.com

Whole Foods Market
   www.wholefoodsmarket.com

ACKNOWLEDGMENTS

Physique 57 Staff: Without each of you, this book would not be a reality. We know that we have the most talented and committed staff imaginable. Every day, you encourage our clients to be the best they can be. Together our future is bright!

Alicia Weihl: Physique 57 has always been a team effort, and you are definitely an MVP. Your creativity, expertise, and pursuit of excellence inspire our clients and staff to reach their fullest potential and become the best version of themselves. Your energy, grace, and perfection make for flawless photos.

Ashley Walker: Thank you for keeping this tremendous project moving in the right direction. From beginning to end, you gave your all to this book, and our readers will reap the benefits of your contribution.

Shelly Knight: Thank you for a great photo shoot. Your tireless smiles, superior strength, and beauty astound us all. Thanks for gracing our pages with your wonderful images.

Karen Keeler: Thank you for gracing the cover of our book with your fabulous figure and for your many contributions to Physique 57.

Carmela Cali: You are completely indispensable. Carmela speed dial will always be close to the top! You are a true artist with many unspoken talents. Carmela = pretty, calm, and ready. You rock!

Sara Beth Turner: You've been a special friend to Physique 57, and it was an honor to collaborate with you. Thank you for capturing the essence of our movements through your lens.

Donna Sonkin: Your passion for healthy eating and living makes you a true gem that shone brightly on this huge endeavor. Thank you for bringing your sparkle, knowledge, and wisdom to our readers.

Bob Otto: Thank you for all your research and your insight into the science behind the magic that is Physique 57.

Ann Campbell: You are the dream collaborator. We are forever grateful to your enduring commitment and dedication to perfecting our inaugural book. You are brilliant and insightful and made writing this book a fun and exciting adventure. Cheers to you!

Diana Baroni at Grand Central: Thank you for your vision and commitment to us and the Physique 57 method. You've been the perfect partner. Thanks also to Amanda Englander for supporting new authors and answering our *many* questions.

Andrea Barzvi at International Creative Management: You've been a great leader and guide through this long journey. We're glad that we've heeded your advice every step of the way. You're a superstar!

Physique 57 Clients, Fans, and Followers: Your stories of triumph and dedication to Physique 57 keep us going on our mission to spread our fitness lifestyle far and wide. Please keep the stories coming. Your enthusiasm and determination inspire us and others to continue on the journey to good health and empowerment.

Special thanks to everyone else who brought this book to life with their wisdom and expertise, including Binky Urban at International Creative Management for taking the meeting and being as excited about Physique 57 as we are; Julie Grau for getting us started in the right direction; and Elizabeth Benson, Elizabeth Lambert, Larissa Bocchi, and Jennifer Goller for pitching in on so many challenging projects—you are amazing teammates.

INDEX

Jennifer's fitness odyssey began in earnest when she opted out of back surgery related to dance injuries and set out to find an effective back- and core-strengthening exercise method. After sampling seemingly every mainstream and New Age class available in New York City, she stumbled across the Lotte Berk Method, cured her back, and reshaped her body. Saddened and desperate after the sudden demise of Lotte, she wrote a business plan and recruited Tanya Becker to quickly ramp up an updated method that would sate the appetite of hundreds of similarly disappointed Lotte Berk acolytes. Jennifer is passionate about her family, business, dance, and exercise. She has found her calling in life—running a world-class service business focused on health and dance-inspired exercise. Jennifer, her supportive husband, and their three young children live in New York City and love to travel around the world.

ABOUT THE AUTHORS

Tanya Becker is the co-founder and senior vice president of programming and training at Physique 57. Prior to creating the Physique 57 method, she trained and taught at the Lotte Berk Method in New York City, where she helped update, refine, and perfect the legendary fitness regimen.

In addition to teaching and training at the Physique 57 studios, Tanya choreographs and performs in the award-winning Physique 57 DVD series. She regularly represents Physique 57 in national media outlets including *The Martha Stewart Show*, the *Today* show, and *Dr. Oz*. She has also been featured in *Vogue, Shape, Redbook, Harper's Bazaar, New York Magazine*, and *People*. She is a well-known personality in the New York fitness scene with a large following of admiring clients. Tanya is tenacious and passionate about her work—she continuously improves and expands the Physique 57 method to keep it perched at the forefront of the fitness industry.

As a trained student of the Luigi Jazz Technique and an accomplished choreographer, Tanya has performed in musicals and live productions around the world and has appeared in many industrials, films, and commercials. She is an ACE (American Council of Exercise) Certified Personal Trainer. Tanya, her husband, and their twins live in Hoboken, New Jersey.

Jennifer Maanavi is the owner, co-founder, and CEO of Physique 57. She has been involved in dance from early childhood, having performed many different genres throughout college. She has a strong Wall Street finance background and earned an MBA from Columbia Business School with high honors. She left Morgan Stanley in 2005 to launch Physique 57.